all about health

AN INTRODUCTION TO HEALTH EDUCATION

Dorothy Baldwin

Oxford University Press 1985

Oxford University Press, Walton Street, Oxford OX2 6DP

Oxford London
New York Toronto Melbourne Auckland
Kuala Lumpur Singapore Hong Kong Tokyo
Delhi Bombay Calcutta Madras Karachi
Nairobi Dar es Salaam Cape Town

and associated companies in
Beirut Berlin Ibadan Mexico City Nicosia

Oxford is a trade mark of Oxford University Press

© Dorothy Baldwin 1985
ISBN 0 19 832719 6

Acknowledgements

The publishers would like to thank the following for permission to reproduce photographs:

Blackwell Biovisual: 22; Camera Press: 162 (right); J. Allan Cash: 162 (left and centre); Charing Cross Hospital: 7; Daily Mail: 106, 146; Down's Children's Association: 145; Patrick Eagar: 156; Richard and Sally Greenhill: 7 ($\times$ 3), 118, 154, 167; B.J. Harris Photography: 130; Institute of Cancer Research/Westminster Hospital/Sir Stanford Cade: 96; Camilla Jessel: 7, 148, 149, 157; Leo Mason: 9; Jessie Ann Matthew: 7; Network/Laurie Sparham: 7; New Scotland Yard: 105; Oral-B: 41; Oxford Mail: 107; Picturepoint: 8; Rosie Potter: 10, 16, 17 (top), 111, 117, 126, 139, 143, 155; Rentokil: 26, 163; Rex Features: 120; Chris Schwarz: 108, 110: St. John's Hospital for Diseases of the Skin: 24 (both), 25; Jenny Thomas: 17 (bottom); C. James Webb: 27; Terry Williams: 99, 101.

Illustrations are by:

Oena Armstrong
Roger Gorringe
Anna Hancock
Hanife Hassan
Kevin Hudson
Viv Mabon
Dave Murray
Jon Riley

Phototypeset by Tradespools Ltd., Frome, Somerset
Printed in Great Britain at the University Press, Cambridge

Preface

All about health brings together in one book all the various health topics considered important for young people today.

However, **All about health** includes far more information than this. Health today is seen largely as a matter of prevention: the prevention of ill-health by sensible decision-making. 'What foods should I eat?' 'How much sleep do I need?' 'How can I cope with negative feelings about myself, or others?' This book is designed to give students the information they need to enable them to make informed choices about their health, both physical and mental. Information on topics such as social welfare and community health is also included to encourage students to think of their health choices in relation to wider social issues.

The book contains five chapters, each of which is broken down into a number of self-contained double-page units. Each unit deals with one particular topic in detail and ends with questions designed to reinforce understanding of the main teaching points. Certain topics, such as family planning and drugs, are covered in more than one unit as the nature of the material requires further explanation and more detailed information. Each unit is intended to stimulate thought and to help develop an enquiring attitude towards health and behaviour. Again and again questions are asked in the 'What do *you* think?' format to encourage a deeper level of discussion and understanding. Throughout, the stress is on a positive attitude to health rather than the dire warnings which have been proven to have little effect. However, where new evidence of destructive health patterns is emerging, this information is also included.

Many of the units contain a 'finding out' section. This is intended to heighten curiosity, and to give students the satisfaction of learning from their own, very simple, research findings. At the end of each chapter is a section of further work. This provides suggestions for learning through direct observation, for practical study, for homework, and for individual project work. Visits to various external agencies are recommended and, where this is not possible, alternative suggestions for study are offered. The questions provide a wide variety of extended work from which the teacher may select, according to the needs and abilities of the students.

The book is designed to be of real value to the teacher in the classroom, especially those working with groups and those tackling the subject of health education for the first time. Medical and technical terms are kept to an absolute minimum and, where used, the explanation is clearly given beside them. Slowly, step by step, best practice in maintaining physical health is spelled out. Adolescence, with its joys, worries, and conflicts, is dealt with in considerable depth. Difficult concepts, such as the relationship between life style and early heart disease, are presented in simple, readily-understood terms The students are encouraged to regard their health in terms of personal choice and personal responsibility. Many units have a self-help section to demonstrate to students that they can face up to and deal with most minor health problems themselves. However, advice is also given on when to visit the doctor and what to do at the surgery.

Chapter 1 looks at all aspects of physical health, with particular emphasis on problems likely to occur in adolescence. Chapter 2, dealing with mental health, covers the emotions and their effect on behaviour. This breaks new ground in health education. But mental illness is increasing at an alarming rate and affects people from all walks of life. The World Health Organization estimates that 40 million people suffer from major mental illness and a further 200 million suffer from minor mental illness: it is considered a major health problem today. As it is now known that much mental illness could have been avoided, the aim of this chapter is largely preventive. Information is given on the basic emotions and how they affect behaviour. Positive attitudes towards conflicting emotions and different methods of coping with them are discussed in some detail. It is hoped that students will gain a better insight into their own and other people's emotional lives, and a better understanding and sympathy for those who do become mentally ill.

The next chapter, 'About the top killers', follows on naturally as many of these are, in part, caused by wrong decision-making in health choices, for example smoking-related diseases such as lung cancer and heart disease. Chapter 4, 'About relationships', contains what might be considered somewhat delicate and sensitive topics. It is hoped that these will be discussed in a delicate and sensitive manner: outside speakers from various named agencies may be used at this stage. However, the units are self-explanatory so that study and written work can be undertaken unaided if desired. The final chapter deals with community health and the medical and social services available – important information students will need in later life. First aid for emergency situations is also covered in this chapter, though students should be encouraged to follow a practical training course in first aid where possible.

Throughout the book, the information is presented and the language especially chosen so as to make the facts readily accessible to all students, whatever their ability. It is hoped that **All about health** will bring to students much-needed information at present lacking in book form in schools, and bring to teachers a reliable reference tool which they can work through with their pupils, gradually building up a coherent, well-constructed body of knowledge in the subject of health education.

Contents

Introduction

The different stages of life

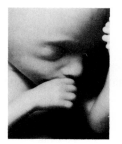

The unborn

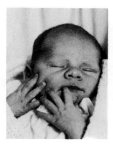

The baby

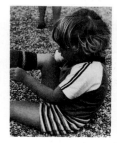

The child

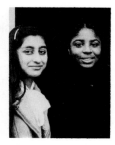

The adolescent

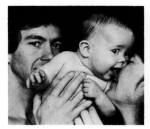

The young adult

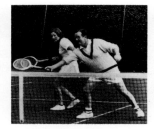

The middle-aged

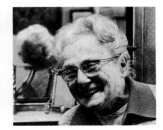

The elderly

The unborn
You begin life as one cell. That single cell divides many times and grows rapidly. It is called an **embryo**. The embryo grows and develops until a new baby is ready to be born. During this time, the mother's health is of great importance. She needs to feel secure and happy with the father. She also needs the support of the medical and social services.

The baby
Babies cannot look after themselves. They cannot keep warm, clean, or dry, nor can they fetch their own food. Babies depend totally on their parents, who must do these things. In turn, parents have support from family and friends. They may need extra help from the community.

The child
Children have learned nearly all their body skills — how to walk, feed themselves, put on clothes, and so on. During this stage, children learn about their society from school and from home. They are also trained in sensible health habits, such as keeping their teeth clean and crossing the road safely.

The adolescent
The adolescent is at the in-between stage; no longer a child but not yet an adult. Some adolescents grow through the teens without any bother. Others find the teens difficult and need extra help from the community.

The young adult
Most young adults are ready for marriage and a family. They are ready to take

their place in society. They become responsible for their own welfare, and the welfare of others too.

The middle-aged
The middle-aged have raised their families and are settled in the community. They are active in health and social welfare: paying taxes, caring for the elderly, looking after grandchildren, and so on.

The elderly
The elderly can look back on a life in which they have played a useful part. They may have health or social troubles which sometimes go with ageing such as heart disease, stiff joints, or loneliness.

On the merry-go-round

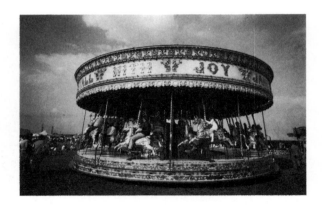

Life is like a merry-go-round. At some stages you will be riding freely (supported by others) and at others you will be working the machinery (giving the support). Each stage in life has different health and social needs from the stage before. The early stages and the last usually have the greatest needs as young and old people are dependent on support from others.

All about health deals mainly with the stage you are at – adolescence. Other stages will be studied where there is information you need. You are already making choices about your future health and welfare. Soon you will be at the stage of choosing to take on the responsibility for others – of giving the support. You need plenty of information to help you make these choices. **All about health** gives you this information and discusses the decisions you will make in five separate chapters:

1 **About physical health** – information on the changes taking place in your body, and how to keep yourself fit and healthy.
2 **About mental health** – information on the changes taking place in your mind and feelings, and how best to help them develop.
3 **About the top killers** – information on the serious health problems of today, and how best to avoid them.
4 **About relationships** – information on now and the future, and discussions on the decisions you are likely to face.
5 **About community health** – information on general health and social welfare which you will need when you are giving the support.

Chapter 1
About physical health

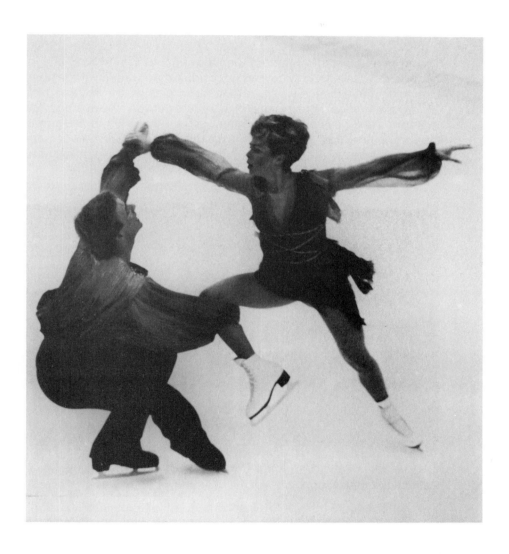

What is adolescence?

Adolescence is the final stage of development before you become an adult. It takes a long time. Not only your body, but your mind and emotions have to grow and develop too. One definition of adolescence is: 'The process or condition of growing up; the period of time between childhood and maturity'.

Average ages

The first signs of starting adolescence are changes in your body shape. You begin to grow taller and to develop your adult shape. The average ages for beginning adolescence are from 10 to 12 for girls, and from 12 to 14 for boys.

You will notice there is a gap of two years between the average ages at which girls and boys begin to develop. Perhaps this is why some girls prefer the company of boys a little older – what do you think? But this age gap between the sexes doesn't last long. By 16 to 17, boys have quickly caught up.

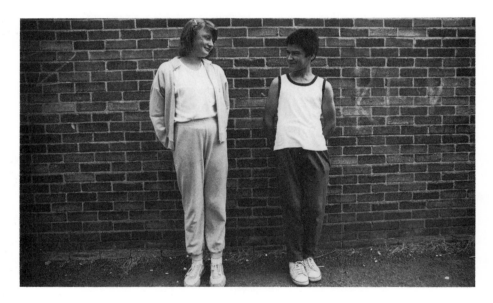

Patterns of development

You start to mature (grow into an adult) according to your family pattern. This means you inherit (get) from your parents the chance to mature at the same time as they did. For example: if your mother didn't start her periods till she was 16, it is likely that you won't; or if your father grew tall by the time he was 14, it is likely that you will too.

Other things also control when you begin to mature. In general, black people mature before white people; people in hot countries before those in cold countries; people with parents in skilled work before those with parents in unskilled work – the reasons why this happens are not fully known. Your general state of health is also likely to affect when you begin to mature. So heredity (family patterns), race, climate, work, and general health all have a part to play in your development.

'Early or late developer?'

Neither. You will notice that the word 'average' is written beside 'ages'. It is important that you understand average ages are just guidelines to work from. They are not rules. There is no need to worry if you do not fit into an average. You are not an early or late developer. You are maturing at the *right time for you*. Remember, there is no such person as a typical teenager. You are changing all the time.

'Key of the door'

In many countries, 18 is the age when you reach your **majority** (come of age). You have full adult rights. You may vote, take out credit facilities, fight for your country, marry and start to raise a family. But in both sexes, bones do not finally harden till you are in your early 20s, and boys often grow taller and stronger long after the age of 18. Also, you are not likely to become an apprentice or a student until you are 18, and that is only the *beginning* of further study.

These points are to remind you that adolescence is to do with the growth and development of the mind, as well as the body and the emotions. You can see it is difficult to give an exact age when adolescence ends and you become an adult.

Finding out:
The average rate of growth in height.

Measure, then work out the average height of the people in your class. Repeat this at the end of the term, then again at the end of the year. Work out the average rate of growth per term.

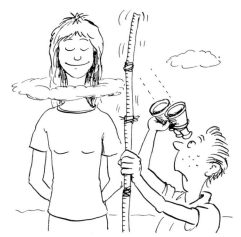

Questions

1 **In your own words, explain what is meant by 'adolescence'.**
2 **What are the average ages for starting adolescence for both sexes?**
3 **What is the time gap between girls and boys? At what age do boys catch up?**
4 **Name four things which control the age at which you begin to mature.**
5 **In some American states, you may fight for your country at 18, but you may not vote, buy alcoholic drinks, or marry without your parents' consent until you are 21. Have a discussion on this.**
6 **Do you think the age of majority should be raised, lowered, or kept at 18? Give reasons for your answer.**

Changes in your body shape

The first part of adolescence is called **puberty**. Puberty is the time when the small compact body of the child begins to change into its adult size and shape. Puberty has to do with physical (body) growth and development. Some of the changes you can see, as they happen on the outside. Others you may not know about as they are internal changes.

The **pituitary** is a small part of your brain which makes **hormones**. Hormones are powerful chemicals which control the proper working of your body. At puberty, your pituitary sends special hormones to your reproductive (sex) organs. Your reproductive organs then start to make the sex hormones which change your body into its adult size and shape.

By the end of puberty, your reproductive organs are working. This means you are capable of having a child. But puberty can end at 13 for a few girls and at 15 for a few boys – they have grown to their full adult size and shape by then. Do you think this is a suitable age to start having a family?

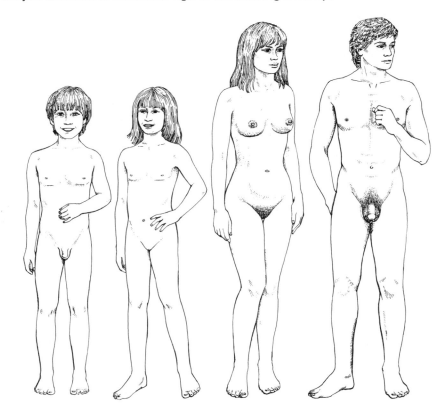

The growth spurt

This is the term for the rapid growth in height which is usually the beginning of puberty. Can you remember suddenly growing out of your clothes and shoes? Notice the different times of growth for girls and for boys. Usually, the growth spurt happens in a particular order.

1 The head, feet, and hands grow to adult size first.
2 Next come the limbs. Your arms and legs grow in length, then in strength.
3 Finally the trunk, which is your body from shoulder to hip, grows to its full adult size and shape.

This order of growing may make you feel awkward for a while. You may think you have huge feet which trip over things, or long arms which keep knocking things aside. Don't worry about feeling clumsy. This stage doesn't last for long. You will soon catch up with yourself and your movements will become graceful and smooth.

Look at the pictures opposite again. Study the body shapes carefully. Notice which of the changes happen to both girls and boys. They are:

1 The growth spurt.
2 Pubic hair which grows on the genitals (the outer part of the sex organs).
3 Axillary hair which grows in the armpits.
4 The reproductive (sex) organs which grow and develop.
5 Skin changes which include new sweat and oil glands.
6 The heart, lungs, muscles, and bones all grow in size and strength.

The different changes

In girls: The figure becomes rounded as the hips widen and the breasts develop. Menstruation (having periods) begins.
In boys: The figure becomes stronger as the chest and back widen, and muscles develop. The voice breaks and nocturnal emissions (producing sperm) begin.
All the changes at puberty will be studied in more detail later on.

Self help
Teenagers who are active – who take a lot of exercise by dancing, gymnastics, or sport – do not go through an awkward clumsy stage. This is because exercise trains the different parts of your body to work smoothly together. If you want to aim for sleek graceful movements right through adolescence, try to make sure you have plenty of exercise.

Questions

1 **In your own words, explain what is meant by 'puberty'.**
2 **What is the name of the chemicals which actually start puberty?**
3 **What is meant by the 'growth spurt'? Name the order in which it happens.**
4 **What is (a) pubic hair and (b) axillary hair?**
5 **Name three changes which happen in both sexes at puberty.**
6 **What can you do to avoid being a bit clumsy during the growth spurt? Why do you think this is likely to work?**
7 **Discuss whether 13 for girls and 15 for boys is a suitable age to start a family.**

Facts about your skin

The surface layer

Rub a wet finger briskly up and down your arm. The tiny bits which come away are dead cells. Millions of dead cells are shed from the surface of your skin every day. They float off into the air, rub off on your clothes and bedding, and are removed when you wash. These dead cells on the surface protect the delicate skin underneath. During the teens, more dead cells are made and the surface of the skin thickens slightly.

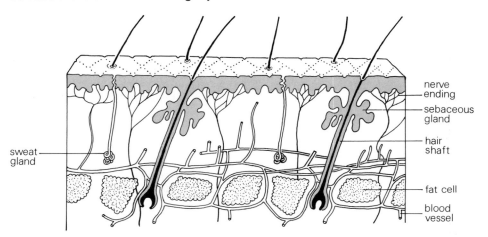

The sweat glands

Adults have about two million sweat glands spread under the surface of the skin. Sweat is mainly water with a little salt and body waste in it. You sweat to keep cool and to keep your body temperature even. Sweating goes on all the time, though you are not aware of it. Between 500 and 700 cc of sweat is lost from your body each day. Heavy sweat, which you are aware of, is caused by such things as exercise, eating hot spicy foods, and feeling anxious or excited. In the teens, new sweat glands under the arms and around the groin begin working. This sweat is slightly thicker and has a musty body odour.

Oily or dry skin?

An oily fluid called **sebum** is made in small glands near the hair shafts. Sebum flows up to the surface of the skin along each tiny hair. Because sebum is an oil, it keeps the hair shiny and the skin smooth and supple. Some people naturally make far more sebum than others. During the teens, people with naturally oily skins sometimes make too much sebum.

Skin colour

Melanin is a pigment (dark colouring) made in special cells under the skin. You inherit your skin colour: a little melanin and you are pale or yellow, more melanin and you are olive, brown, or black. Melanin protects the skin from the harsh rays of the sun by making more pigment. Dark people go darker but, as melanin takes time to be made, pale people often 'burn' instead of getting a tan.

Melanin also forms the colour of your eyes and hair. As people get older, less melanin is made. This is why hair may grow white and eye colour fade. Even during the teens, you may find one or two white hairs! Freckles are the result of pigment cells being clumped together, instead of evenly spread out. If you have freckles *and* red hair, it is likely your skin will burn in sunlight.

Sunbathing

Sunbathing ages the skin, making it thick, wrinkly, and leathery. But the fashion for a tan does not seem likely to change quickly, and sunlight does have healing effects on skin conditions such as acne (pp. 22–3). If you wish to sunbathe, do it in short stages. It takes four days to produce melanin and a week for the skin cells to grow thicker. Start with fifteen minutes, then double the time over the next few days. In between, keep your skin covered up. Suntan preparations are helpful but you must follow the instructions carefully.

Sunburn

The skin turns hot, red, and painful. There is burning and itching for a day or more. It takes about a week for the burned skin to blister and peel away. Badly-burned people may get painful headaches and spells of dizziness and sickness.

SKIN TYPE	PROTECTION NEEDED	PROTECTION FACTOR	COPPERTONE PRODUCT
Dark/ Tans Easily No Burns	Minimum	2	'Lite' Oil or Cream
Normal Tans easily Rarely Burns	Minimum	2	'Lite' Oil or Cream
Normal Tans Moderately Some Burns	Moderate	4	Lotion or Cream
Fair Burns Easily	Extra	6	Lotion or Cream
Sensitive Burns Easily	Extra	8	Water-Resistant Lotion
Very sensitive Always burns	Maximum (Sun Block)	15	Super Shade 15 Lotion

Self help

If you do burn: drink plenty of water; stay right out of sunlight; use cool water to reduce the pain and calamine lotion to soothe the skin.

Finding out:

About protection factors in suntan products.

Collect leaflets which advertise different suntan preparations. Study and then make notes on what is said about protection factors. Find out which one you think will suit you best.

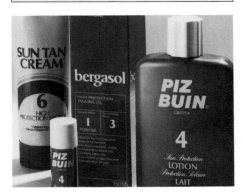

Questions

1 **What happens to the dead cells on the surface of the skin?**
2 **What is sweat? How many sweat glands are there in an adult body?**
3 **How much sweat that you are not aware of do you lose each day?**
4 **What is sebum? Describe its function.**
5 **Write a short paragraph, explaining how to avoid getting sunburnt.**

Hair and nails

Hair and nails are made in the skin, from a hard substance called **keratin**. Hair is dead, but grows about 1 cm a month from the live root. It lasts from two to ten years, falls out and is replaced. You inherit hair type, colour, and thickness. A tendency to early baldness also runs from father to son. As yet, no cream or lotion will cure baldness or make hair grow any thicker.

Head hair

The appearance of your hair 'says' something about you. During a mood swing (p. 82), don't rush to change your style if you think you might regret it. Your hair should be washed frequently or it will smell unfresh and look unattractive. Remember, too, to wash your brush and comb at the same time. Hair may split or break at the ends. Check this is not caused by perms, bleaches, or straighteners. Cut the damaged ends off and give the hair a rest.

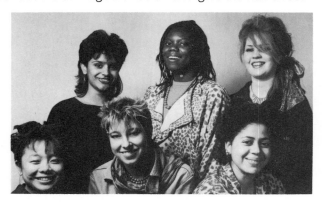

Dandruff

Dandruff is the dead skin cells which flake off the scalp. Dandruff is harmless; you cannot catch it, nor pass it on. But it looks unattractive. If your hair is oily, try a dandruff treatment shampoo. Otherwise, brush well to remove the dandruff flakes and to bring more sebum down the hair shaft.

The scalp can get infected if too much oil clings to dandruff. The skin of your head becomes red, sore, and itchy. If you scratch, the patches ooze and may spread along the hairline. Go to the doctor for advice and treatment.

Body hair

The lips, eyelids, palms, and soles of the feet are hairless. The rest of the body is hairy. You may have fine down which can hardly be seen, or clumps here and there, or a thick matted rug. Try not to worry about body hair – like yourself the way you are. Girls with hairy legs are *just* as womanly; boys with hairy shoulders are *not* more manly.

For girls: In some countries, underarm hair is considered attractive. In other countries, it is not. If you do remove underarm hair, take care not to damage the skin. Boils and other infections can easily start this way. Keep your equipment scrupulously clean.

Face hair

For boys, beard growth can start in the mid teens; often it is later. You may get a slight rash just before the hair appears. After shaving, wipe the razor with antiseptic (any lotion which kills germs). Some after-shave products have astringents which make the skin sore or toughen it too much. A beard saves shaving time, but check it stays free of debris and food.

Nails

Nails begin to grow near the first joint of your fingers where the cells are very sensitive. If you damage this area, the cells over-react and produce extra layers so there is a thick horny lump. A blow near the cuticle (nail edge) causes a blood blister which grows out in the three to six months of average nail growth. A **whitlow** is an infection of the skin at the side of the nail. It must be treated by a doctor to stop the germs spreading under the nail.

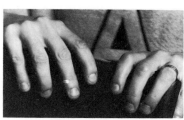
Bitten nails look ugly.

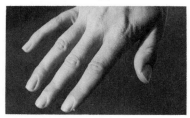
Well-kept nails.

Care of the nails

1 Brittle nails, which flake, chip, or peel, should be cut right down with nail clippers or sharp scissors. Cut in small straight snips to avoid bending the rest of the nail. Emery boards are not suitable for brittle nails. The filing action can make things worse.

2 Cuticles should not need to be pushed back. Proper drying of the hands, from the tips downwards, should keep them in place. But if you do push them back, take care not to break open the skin. Hang-nails (bits of torn cuticle) must not be bitten or pulled off. Cut them down close to the skin. If the raw edges keep snagging, cover with plaster while they heal.

3 Nail-biting can be a comfort habit left over from childhood, or a way of getting rid of tension. If you do bite your nails, try to decide why. If it is a comfort habit, you should be able to stop quite soon. But habits caused by tense feelings can be more difficult to stop. You will have to learn to cope with tension before your nails can grow (p. 69).

Questions

1 **Where are hair and nails made, and from what?**
2 **What advice would you give to a friend whose hair was split at the ends?**
3 **Give three reasons why hair should be washed frequently.**
4 **How would you treat dandruff in (a) oily hair and (b) dry hair?**
5 **Name the parts of the body which are hairless.**
6 **Explain how you would take care of brittle nails.**
7 **What is a 'hang-nail'? How would you treat it?**
8 **Write a short essay, discussing care of the hair and nails.**

Keeping clean and healthy

Germs

There is a saying: 'Adam had 'em'. We share our bodies with millions of **microbes**. These are living creatures so tiny they can only be seen under a microscope. Microbes are also in the world around us, in the air we breathe and the things we touch. Some microbes are helpful. We use them to make bread and cheese. The microbes which cause disease are called **germs**.

Body defences

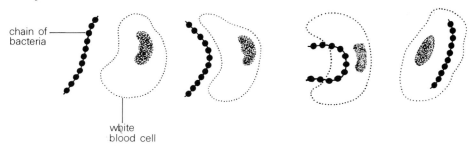

chain of bacteria

white blood cell

White blood cells attack and destroy invading germs.

The skin acts as a barrier to stop germs getting in. When the skin is broken open, there is always a risk of infection. White blood cells and special chemicals rush to destroy the invading germs. During the battle, a lot of **pus** is made. Pus is a mixture of dead and still-fighting germs, and dead and still-fighting white blood cells. It is very infectious.

    Your body defences also control the germs which live inside you. When you are healthy, these germs do you no harm. An example of this is the cold germ which lives in the breathing passages. The cold germ will flare up when you are run down – not eating properly, not having enough sleep, exercise, or fresh air. (You can also catch a cold from another person's sneezes and coughs.)

Body lubricants

Machines need oils, fluids, and creams to keep their parts working smoothly and free of dust and grime. Your body makes its own fluids or **lubricants**:

1 Tears constantly wash the eyes, keeping them clean and damp.
2 Wax oils the ear tunnels and traps any dust which enters.
3 Mucus, which is a thin slippery fluid, keeps the air passages clean.
4 The genitals have their own special lubricants . . . and so on.

Body odour

Sweat, even underarm sweat, is nice when it is fresh – a special 'you' smell. All your body lubricants smell nice. But if sweat remains for long on your skin, germs start to breed on it. This is what produces unpleasant body odour. You can tell this is so because the smell disappears as soon as you wash. During the teens, there may be times of extra sweating caused by unsettled feelings. Damp palms, clammy feet, or feeling sticky all over can happen when you feel embarrassed or insecure (not sure of yourself).

Keeping clean and healthy

Germs breed best in moist places that are not often washed. If you keep your skin clean, they have little time to breed. A good diet, plus plenty of exercise, sleep, and fresh air will keep you healthy and fit. Your body defences need all the help they can get in the battle against germs. When you are clean and healthy, you have a **natural resistance** to disease.

More about germs

Viruses are the smallest germs. Some of the diseases they cause are the common cold, influenza (flu), measles, mumps, and chicken pox. The germs of **bacteria** are larger than viruses. They cause such diseases as whooping cough, food poisoning, and boils. Skin troubles such as athlete's foot (p. 24) are caused by a **fungus**, a mould which can grow on skin.

Self help
Take care of any break in the skin. Cuts and grazes can be held under cold running water to wash out any germs. Small cuts heal quickly if they are left open to the fresh air. The ultra-violet rays in sunlight kill many bacteria. Larger cuts need to be covered with a plaster while the healing scab forms. The plaster stops new germs getting in, and prevents your wound from infecting other people.

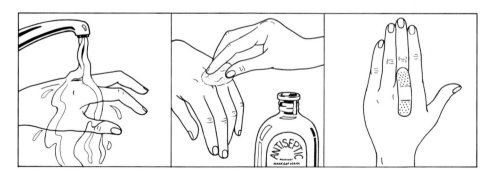

Questions

1 **Name three kinds of germs which live on the body and cause disease. Beside each, list the diseases they cause.**
2 **What is pus? Say why it is very infectious.**
3 **What is meant by 'body lubricants'? Name three kinds and state their function.**
4 **In your own words, explain what causes unpleasant body odour.**
5 **Explain how you would treat a small break in the skin. Give reasons for this treatment.**

Hygiene during the teens

Some reasons for extra care over hygiene in the teens are:

1 The extra dead cells made on the top layer of skin.
2 The newly-working sweat glands in the armpits and groin.
3 The extra sweating which may happen because of unsettled feelings.
4 The extra sebum which is made, especially in people with oily skins.

General attention

Wash the whole body regularly to remove dust and grime, and to stop germs breeding on the extra body oils and fluids made in the teens.

If possible, try to take a shower after exercise.

Clothes in contact with the skin – underwear, shirts, socks – should be washed regularly.

Special attention

Cleanse the face carefully to guard against acne spots (p. 22).

Hands should be washed after using the toilet and before preparing or eating food to guard against passing on germs.

Thorough washing of the armpits and groin helps to guard against unpleasant odours.

Feet should be washed to guard against fungus infection (p. 24) and unpleasant odour.

Your basic tools are: hot water, soap, a nail-brush, and a towel.

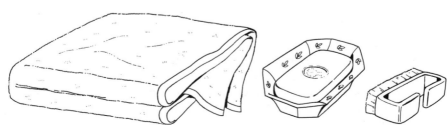

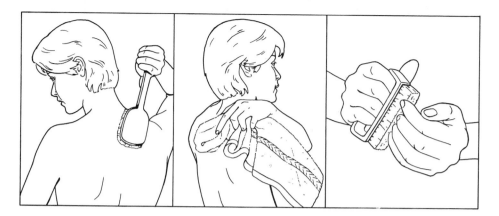

1 Hot water melts body oils, soap breaks them down.
2 Both remove germs, dead cells, sweat, dust, and grime from the skin.
3 If your skin is oily, scrub your back and shoulders with a brush.
4 Rinse your skin thoroughly with clear running water.
5 Dry briskly with the towel to remove the dead cells.
6 Scrub nails and dirty knuckles with the nail-brush.
7 Do not poke inside your ears but make sure the outer parts are clean.

Is your hygiene patchy?

A few people have uneven hygiene. They may spend hours in the bath, and then put on soiled clothes. Or they may wash their face carefully, but forget to clean their nose. Check that your hygiene isn't patchy. Guard against waxy ears, a grubby neck, a dirty nose, unwashed hair, sweaty feet, grimy nails, or mossy teeth in an otherwise perfectly clean body. Build a routine so you don't forget one particular place. Help yourself to be healthy and clean.

Anti-perspirants and deodorants

Nowadays, most underarm creams or lotions contain both of these. An anti-perspirant cuts down sweating by closing some of the pores. A deodorant cuts down odour as it contains antiseptic to stop germs breeding. But neither can give complete protection. Don't worry or feel you are over-sweaty if they don't work. It is up to you whether you use one, or whether you stick with hot water and soap.

Questions

1 **Copy out the four reasons why extra care over hygiene is needed in the teens.**
2 **Why are hot water and soap so important?**
3 **Explain what is meant by 'anti-perspirants and deodorants'.**
4 **A young teenager comes to stay with you and goes to bed without washing. Write a short essay, describing how you would explain the importance of hygiene in such a way that your teenage guest promptly becomes clean.**

What is acne?

The word acne means 'an eruption on the skin'. Acne starts with spots breaking out on the face. The most usual places are the forehead, the sides of the nose, and around the jaw and the chin. Spots can spread to the shoulders, chest, and back. Acne may start in the mid-teens, and is more usual in people with oily skins. Over half of all boys aged 14 to 18 have some acne. It is slightly less common in girls, though more spots are likely to appear around the time of their periods.

Acne starts with spots

Spots can be whiteheads, blackheads, pimples, or angry-looking lumps under the skin. If you are unlucky, you may get all of these at the same time. The change of hormones at adolescence often causes more oil and sweat to be made. The oil and sweat form a greasy film on the surface of the skin. The extra dead cells also made during the teens mixes with the greasy film. These three things *plus* the dirt in the air around you form a perfect breeding ground for germs.

You may remember that the skin thickens slightly during the teens. This can block off the passage of oil to the surface. The trapped sebum hardens, forming a solid little plug with a dark top. Or it may become infected and form a pimple or whitehead. The angry-looking lumps under the skin can be infected sweat or oil glands. The pores to the surface of the skin are blocked.

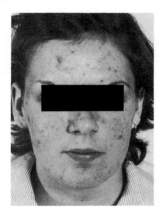

Spreading the infection

The trouble with spots is that they are so satisfying to pick! Many people cannot resist the temptation. They settle down in front of the mirror for a long squeezing session. Other people touch their spots absent-mindedly. While talking or studying, they finger one spot after another. They carry germs back and forward all over their face. The spot-picker and the spot-toucher actually infect their own skins!

If you are one of these people, remember that a spot is full of germs. So are your hands, your fingernails, the dirt in the air, and the greasy film on your skin. Try never to touch spots, no matter how awful you imagine they look. Other people don't notice them half as much as you think.

Is acne dangerous?

Acne is the word used to describe a serious outcrop of spots. But there is no danger to your general health. When your hormones settle down, acne will clear up – usually by the early 20s. As a single acne spot heals, it leaves a purplish mark which soon fades. But very infected spots – often those which have been squeezed or touched – can take weeks to heal and may leave tiny permanent scars.

Keeping acne at bay

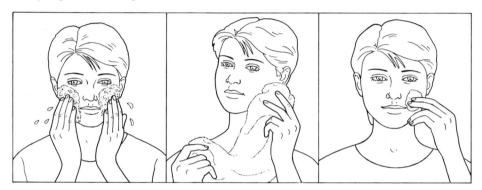

1 Wash your face thoroughly, at least twice a day to keep it really clean.
2 Use an unscented soap as some perfumes irritate the skin.
3 Well-washed hands are better than face cloths as these often hold germs.
4 Rinse with scoops of cold water as this helps to close the pores.
5 Brisk drying brings blood to the surface and tones up the skin.
6 For infected areas and delicate skin, pat dry gently instead.
7 Dab spots with antiseptic lotion on clean cotton wool. Remember to use a fresh piece for each spot or you will spread the infection.

Self help

Sunlight often helps to clear up spots; get outdoors when you can. Diet is often blamed for teenage spots, especially chocolate and fried foods. This has not been proved, but too much of these foods is not good for you in other ways (pp. 42–3). Drink plenty of water as this really does improve the skin. If self help fails and you think your acne is getting worse, go to the doctor.

Questions

1 **What does the word 'acne' mean?**
2 **Where are the most usual places for teenage spots?**
3 **Name the three things which make up the greasy film on the skin.**
4 **What else is added to make a perfect breeding ground for germs?**
5 **Why do you think washing the face thoroughly is so important?**
6 **Spots are also caused by the skin thickening slightly during the teens. In your own words, explain why.**
7 **'Some people actually infect their own skins.' Discuss in what ways this is done.**

Some skin troubles

Boils

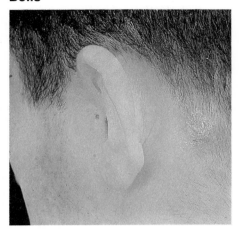

Boils are caused by germs which infect the roots of hairs. They grow much larger than acne spots and should not be confused with them. The whitish matter inside a boil is called **pus**. Pus is full of germs. The boil grows hard and large; it rises until it is ready to burst. This may take about a week and the whole area feels tender and sore.

Self help

Anyone can get a boil at any stage of life. They sometimes start where there is friction, on the neck if your collar rubs, on the bottom if your trousers are too tight. Hold cotton wool soaked in hot salty water over the boil every few hours. This helps to reduce the tenderness and pain. *Do not squeeze the boil.* It should be left to burst in its own time. Clean the area with antiseptic lotion and wash your hands thoroughly. Go to the doctor if you are worried, or if you keep getting boils.

Impetigo

The germs of impetigo are passed by contact: by touching things which are already infected. The germs get in where the skin is broken. Cracked lips, the corners of the mouth, and spots which have been picked are the usual places. Little 'weepy' blisters appear. They dry and form a golden shiny crust. The crust falls off without leaving a scar.

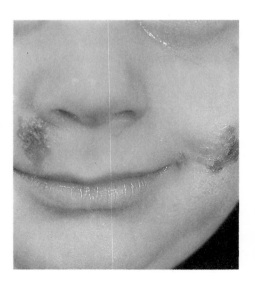

Self help

Go to the doctor for treatment. At home, take *extra* hygiene precautions, especially when preparing food. Impetigo is very infectious in schools or groups of young people. The doctor may tell you to stay at home for a few days.

Ringworm

There are no worms in ringworm! It is a fungus infection (p. 19) of the skin which grows outwards into a ring. Ringworm of the scalp is more common in young children. **Athlete's foot** (fungus between and under the toes) and **ringworm of the upper leg** are the more usual kinds of fungus infection in the teens.

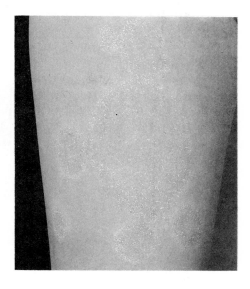

Ringworm is infectious and there are often outbreaks of it in schools, colleges, and sports clubs. It is passed by contact – sharing towels and sports gear, particularly shoes. It can also be picked up from the wooden boards and bare floors of gyms and changing rooms. It is more common in boys and spreads more rapidly in warm weather. Some men have athlete's foot long after they have ceased playing sport.

Self help for athlete's foot
The skin between the toes turns red, flaky, and itchy. When the feet are damp, the infected patches turn white and soggy, then peel. Buy an antifungal powder from the chemist. Use it exactly according to the instructions. At the same time, take extra care to keep your feet clean and dry. Socks, stockings, and tights must be changed daily and the inside of damp shoes dusted with talcum powder. If it does not clear up, go to the doctor for a stronger anti-fungal cream.

Self help for ringworm of the upper leg
This can take a long time to clear up. Be patient and thorough. A typical patch can grow from 5 to 7 cm down the inside of the thigh. Buy anti-fungal ointment and powder from the chemist. Remember to sprinkle trousers, underwear, and pyjamas with the powder daily. If new patches appear or if you feel it is not clearing up, go to your doctor.

Questions

1 **Describe how a boil develops.**
2 **Who gets boils? Where are they likely to start?**
3 **How are the germs of impetigo passed? What advice would you give to a friend about hygiene?**
4 **Describe the way impetigo develops.**
5 **What is ringworm? Name two kinds which are common in the teens.**
6 **How is ringworm passed? Name three things you can do to avoid catching ringworm.**
7 **In public swimming baths, there are heavily-chlorinated pools to step into before you enter the main pool. What infection does this help to prevent?**

Fleas, lice, and scabies

Fleas

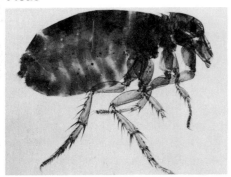

The human flea feeds on blood. It has two horny tubes instead of a mouth. The tubes pierce the skin and blood is sucked up one tube while saliva is poured down the other. Inside the saliva is a special substance which stops your blood clotting while the insect feeds. It is this substance which causes the flea 'bite' – a raised bump which itches.

Self help

It can be difficult to catch a flea! It has powerful legs and can jump long distances. When not feeding, it hides close to the skin or in underclothes, nightwear, sheets, or blankets. Strip off. Put your clothes and bedding in a separate laundry bag. Plunge right down in the bath, with even your head under water (briefly), as the flea may hop up and hide in your hair. If the family pet has fleas, treat it with flea powder.

Lice

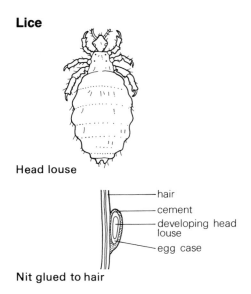

Head louse

hair
cement
developing head louse
egg case

Nit glued to hair

Lice actually live on the human body. They have curved claws to give them a firm grip on the hair. The head louse is common among children, though older people may also catch them. Pubic lice or 'crabs' live in the pubic hair (p. 13). The female louse lays about sixty eggs called **nits** each month. She glues each nit to the hair with a strong cement. It takes about a week for the nit to hatch out, and it is fully grown in three weeks.

Lice cause intense itching. Anyone can catch them. It is now thought that regular combing of the hair will cut down the risk.

Self help

Like fleas, lice are blood-suckers, but they cannot jump. They crawl from person to person where the hair is in close contact. In rare cases, the head louse is passed by borrowing brushes and combs. The head louse can be treated with a nit comb and special lotion bought from the chemist. The treatment has to be repeated until all the nits are removed. Pubic lice, however, should be treated at the special clinic (p. 141). They are passed during sexual contact and it is wise to check for any further damage.

Scabies

Scabies is an infestation of tiny blood-sucking creatures called **mites**. The female burrows under the skin, usually where it is thin, damp, or folded – under the breasts in women; on the inner wrists, the genitals, between the fingers and toes and on the sides of the feet in either sex. She lays her eggs at the end of the 'tunnel', which can be seen from the surface as a thin dark line. In a few days, the eggs hatch and the mites crawl out and begin to feed. They mate with the male mites which stay on the surface of the skin, and so the life cycle begins all over again.

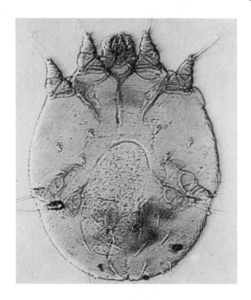

Self help

Scabies cause intense itching. *The skin must not be scratched.* Scratching helps to spread scabies, and breaks open the skin. Scabies are treated by painting the area with a special lotion bought from the chemist. Follow the instructions carefully. A hot bath and scrub is needed before and after treatment. The treatment must be repeated to make sure *all* the eggs under the skin are destroyed. Clothing worn during this time should be boiled, or painted with the lotion, or left for three weeks, by which time the scabies will have died.

Scabies can be passed by infected bedding or clothes. But the most usual way is by direct skin contact.

Health and hygiene

1 Fleas, lice, and scabies are not a direct threat to health.
2 However, they do cause intense itching, and they break open the skin.
3 Wherever the skin is broken, there is a risk of germs entering.
4 Pubic lice and scabies of the genital area should be treated at the special clinic to check that no further damage has been done.
5 Blood-suckers thrive best in damp, dark places on the body. With any infection, extra care with hygiene is essential.
6 Go to the doctor if there is any doubt about what is causing the itching, or if the self-help treatment is not working.

Questions

1 **Explain the way in which a flea feeds.**
2 **List the different ways in which fleas, lice, and scabies are passed.**
3 **'It is pointless to blame the child or the school for an outbreak of head lice.' Do you agree, or disagree? Give reasons for your answer.**
4 **Describe the life cycle of the scabies mite.**
5 **Copy out the health and hygiene points.**

Bones and feet

Bones grow quickly during the teens (p. 12). The average age when growth stops is 16 for girls and 17¾ for boys. Any height from 140 cm (4' 7") to 200 cm (6' 7") is perfectly normal. It is thought that the hormone for growing works while you sleep; so eat well, exercise every day, and have plenty of sleep.

How bones harden

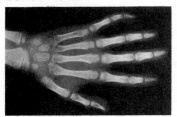

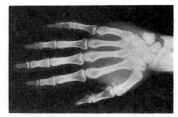

Child's hand   Adult's hand

Notice the different amounts of bone. **Cartilage** is a tough substance which doesn't show up in X-rays – feel it in your nose and ears. Babies and children have a lot of cartilage in their bones, which makes them 'bendy'. Gradually, cartilage hardens into bone and bones are fully hardened by the early 20s. Old people's bones may become dry and brittle, and snap easily. Never hurry an old person in case they fall. Their bones take a long time to mend.

Joints

Joints are where two or more bones meet – they allow movement. Joints are held together by tough **ligaments**, and kept well lubricated to stop any friction. A torn ligament is not unusual among athletes. Being 'double-jointed' simply means that you have larger ligaments, so the joint has further movement.

Swollen joints in old people are caused by bone and cartilage wearing out. Between the knobbly bones of your spine are **discs** of cartilage to stop friction and act as shock-absorbers. You know they are important if you land, jarringly, on your heels! Never pull a chair away as someone is about to sit down. It is very dangerous, and not at all funny.

Damage to bones

When a bone breaks, it is called a **fracture**. Any bone will break with very rough treatment. Collar bones and limb bones are top of the list. If you think there may be a fracture, *do not move the injured part*. Call a doctor or an ambulance. A fracture must be 'set' and then firmly wrapped in plaster so that the ends of the broken bones can grow together again.

Self help for sprains

Have you ever twisted your ankle or turned back your wrist? There is pain and swelling. You wonder if it is a **sprain** – a torn ligament or other damage to the joint. Rest your foot on a stool, or your arm in a sling, and wrap damp cloths around the injured joint. If the pain and swelling don't go down after a couple of hours, go to the hospital for an X-ray.

Care of the feet

Babies have lovely feet with straight toes. Many adults don't. The problem usually starts in the teens, especially for girls. If you remember that bones take a long time to harden, you can guess at the harm done by badly-fitting shoes. High heels and pointed toes worn too early are particularly damaging as they force growing bones into strange and unnatural positions. You may get crooked toes, or corns (which are hardened skin cells), or bunions (outgrowths of bone) – or all three. Nearly all corns, bunions, and crooked toes are the triumph of vanity over common sense!

1 During the teens buy shoes which allow room for growth.
2 Have *both* feet measured, as one foot is often larger than the other.
3 Try on both shoes, walk around, stand on tip-toe. Shoes must be comfortable.
4 Never try to 'break in' shoes which pinch or rub. They will break your feet in first, causing ugly bunions and corns.

Foot hygiene

Sweaty feet must be washed often to cut down the risk of athlete's foot (p. 24). Socks, tights, or stockings can be washed through at the same time. Pad around in bare feet or open sandals when possible; leave boots unlaced or unzipped when not in use. Check under toe-nails for debris, dead skin cells, and dirt and remove it. Do this regularly and any odour should disappear.

Toe-nails

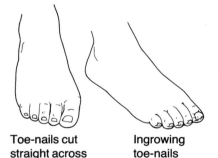

Toe-nails cut
straight across

Ingrowing
toe-nails

These should always be cut straight across. Do this after a bath when the toe-nails are soft. Toe-nails which are too long grow into claws which buckle under the toes. Toe-nails which are cut too short at the sides grow into the skin. This can cause a painful condition called 'ingrowing toe-nails'.

Questions

1 **What is the average age when bone growth stops for (a) girls, (b) boys?**
2 **Write a few lines about cartilage.**
3 **What is a fracture? Explain the treatment for it.**
4 **You twist an ankle and cannot decide whether it is sprained or not. What self-help treatment would you try?**
5 **Write a short essay, discussing the care of the feet.**
6 **Name three things which can be done to avoid foot odour.**

Muscles and posture

Muscles increase in size and length during the teens. The strength of muscles almost doubles between the ages of 12 and 16. Athletic ability improves enormously in boys. In some girls, it peaks at 13 or 14, and then declines. The reasons why this happens are not really known.

How muscles work

Muscles pull on bone to move you. They work in pairs. The **biceps** muscle contracts to pull your lower arm up, then the **triceps** muscle contracts to pull it down. Messages travel along nerves from your brain, telling muscles to contract. Find out how fast these messages can travel by drumming a finger up and down on the desk. If the nerve is damaged, the muscle receives no message. Though it is perfectly healthy, it cannot move. This is called **paralysis**.

Muscles are attached to bones by cords called **tendons**. Tendons are so strong that a violent jerk can snap off a piece of bone before a tendon snaps. But tendons do get torn, and have to be stitched back.

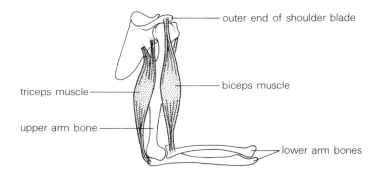

Muscle tone

Relax your hand on the desk. Notice the position of your fingers. They are neither stretched out stiffly nor clenched into a fist. This is because muscles never completely relax. They are always in a slight state of tension called **muscle tone**. Muscle tone keeps you ready for instant action. It also keeps your body in an upright **posture** without you thinking about it. An unconscious person loses muscle tone and becomes a 'dead' weight.

Posture

Are you being warned by adults about slouching or stooping? Remember that bad posture can lead to health problems now and in the future.

1 Head poked forward – tension headache. Early double chin.
2 Shoulders hunched – cramped chest, droopy breasts. Breathing troubles later.
3 Back slumped – slight hunch. Backache, slipped disc, pot-belly later.
4 Weight on one hip – backache. Varicose veins, pot-belly later.

The teens are the 'make or break' years for posture. Muscle and bone develop together, giving support and shape to your growing adult frame. Bad posture causes curving of the bones, especially the spine, and muscles have to adapt to the new altered shape. Over the years, this deformity will become fixed. You shouldn't need to be warned about posture. Common sense tells you how important it is.

Standing posture

a b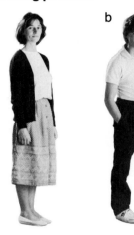

Head is squarely on the shoulders, chin not up nor down.
Chest is raised and shoulders are spread wide, not pulled back.
Stomach is tucked in so weight is balanced evenly over hips.
Knees are straight, but not pulled stiffly back.
Feet are squarely on the ground so body weight is evenly balanced.

Sitting posture

c 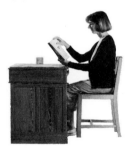 b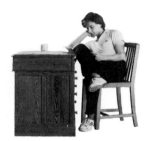

Sitting should be like standing from the hips up. Hips should be well back and supported by the chair. Feet should be squarely on the floor. If you cross your legs, cross them at the ankle only. Shoulder blades were not made for sitting on, so don't use them to support your weight!

Questions

1 **Explain simply how muscles work.**
2 **What is muscle tone and why is it important?**
3 **What health problems happen (a) now and (b) later due to bad posture?**
4 **Why is it so important to develop good posture in the teens?**
5 **Check your posture in a full-length mirror. How do you look? How could you improve? Turn sideways and check your tummy is well tucked in.**
6 **Study pictures b and d. Write a few lines explaining in what ways each posture is incorrect.**

Keeping fit

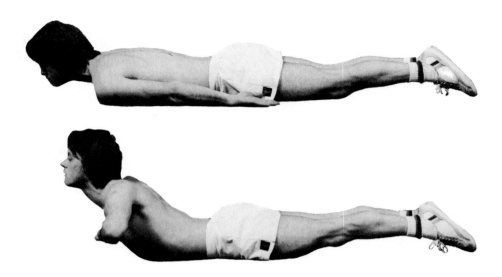

Exercises for strength

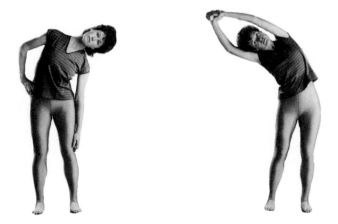

Exercises for suppleness

Vigorous exercise is any series of movements you do which makes you sweaty, breathless, and aware that your heart is pounding. During vigorous exercise you breathe more deeply to get oxygen into your lungs, your heart beats more rapidly to pump the blood rich in oxygen to your muscles, and you sweat more heavily to get rid of the extra heat. All this not only tones up your muscles but is a complete tonic for your whole body – making it fit, healthy, and strong.

Vigorous exercise is important throughout life, but especially so while you are still developing. It is essential for:

1 **Strength** Muscles actually waste away if they are not used. Vigorous exercise increases their size and builds up their strength.
2 **Suppleness** If joints are not regularly stretched to their full extent, they stiffen. Exercise will help you move with grace and ease.

3 **Stamina** Muscles need to keep on going, not collapse after one quick burst of effort. You build up physical stamina by regular exercise.

4 **Safety** Vigorous exercise gets rid of tense, anxious, or angry feelings. You feel pleasantly tired, more relaxed about problems, and less likely to be upset.

Athletic ability

Some people are naturally athletic. They move with physical grace and are good at sports. Others have to work hard. Though they improve their body skills, they never quite manage that lovely graceful ease. This is the way people are – naturally different. But it would be a mistake to give up exercise just because you are not naturally athletic.

Different skills

Remember, part of your awkwardness may be due to the growth spurt (p. 12). Whatever the cause, there are different kinds of exercise to suit people's different body skills and personalities. If you dislike competitive sports, have you thought of jogging or cycling, swimming or rowing, dancing or aerobics, or simply exercising in the privacy of your room?

Cramps and stitches

Oxygen and food are 'burned' in the muscles to give you energy. If you over-exercise, your muscles run short of oxygen. You feel the pain of a stitch or cramp. Rest, and the pain will disappear. Another kind of cramp starts if you swim after eating a large meal. This is always dangerous, especially if you are out of your depth. A severe cramp will 'unknot' if you stretch the muscle right out. This is painful, but it works.

Finding out:
Your breathing rate during vigorous exercise.

Using a stop watch, time how many breaths you take a minute while sitting quietly. Then time yourself after two minutes of vigorous exercise. (This should not be done by people with breathing problems.)
Copy the chart and fill in your results.

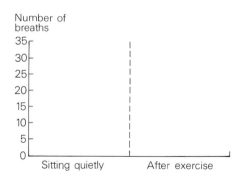

Questions

1 **Give the definition of 'vigorous exercise'.**
2 **In what ways does vigorous exercise act as a complete tonic?**
3 **Copy out the four points which explain the importance of vigorous exercise.**
4 **Only a few of the different kinds of exercise are mentioned here. Think up at least three more and write a sentence about each one.**

Lungs and breathing

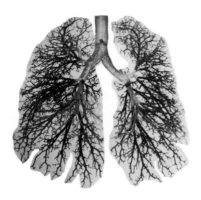

If your lungs were stretched out, they would cover the area of a tennis court. They begin under your shoulders and go down to the end of your ribs, front and back. They are made of tubes rather like the branches of a tree which get smaller and smaller till they end in tiny air sacs. Here **oxygen** is passed into the blood and the waste gas **carbon dioxide** is passed back. Before air reaches the sacs, it is cleaned, warmed, and moistened – if you breathe through your nose.

The safe passage of air

It is warm and damp in your nose, and there are hairs to trap dust and germs. The air passage or **windpipe** is in front of the food passage or **gullet**. Food must not go down the windpipe. A flap slides over the top when you swallow. Sometimes the flap doesn't close quickly enough – for example, if you talk or laugh while trying to swallow. Huge racking coughs will force the food out.

First aid

If someone is choking, you must act quickly. Brain cells die within four minutes of being without oxygen. Usually, choking is caused by a lump of half-chewed food which is stuck in the windpipe. If you can see it, try hooking it out with your finger. Turn the person so the head is below the knees. Banging on the back is likely to bring the food up.

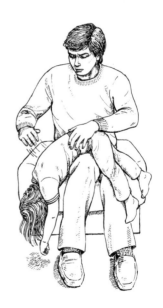

Sweeping the air passages clean

Lining the passages are cells which make a thin sticky liquid, **mucus**. There are also millions of tiny hairs which ripple upwards, twelve times a second, night and day. Any dirt in the air sticks to the mucus which is rippled up to your throat. If it is infected, you cough it out as **catarrh**. Otherwise it is swallowed.

This clever, simple way of sweeping the air passages clean is damaged by smoking (p. 98).

The voice box or Adam's Apple is also in the windpipe. In the teens, the vocal cords grow longer in boys. The voice 'breaks', and there is a deeper pitch or tone. Women and children have shorter vocal cords, so the sounds they make are higher in pitch.

How you breathe

The **diaphragm** is a sheet of muscle between the chest and the lower trunk. It lowers and air is drawn in. It rises and air is forced out. During exercise, the rib muscles also help by pulling the ribs up and outwards so that more air is drawn in. The more exercise you take, the more your lung capacity (how much air you can hold) will increase. A baby breathes about 45 times a minute; a 6-year-old about 25 times; a 15 to 25-year-old about 18 times, which is close to the adult average of 16 to 18. Breathing rates increase again with old age.

Coughs and colds

A cough is a sudden clearing of the air passages. But coughing with sneezing and a blocked or runny nose means you have a cold. As yet, there is no cure for the common cold. Help it to clear up quickly by checking your diet and the amount of exercise, sleep, and fresh air you are getting. Use a handkerchief to stop germs being shot into the air and infecting other people.

Finding out:
Your lung capacity.

Fill a 5-litre plastic bottle with water. Turn it upside-down in a basin of water. Put a rubber tube through the neck. Take a *normal* breath. Blow out down the tube. Mark how much water has been blown out of the bottle and into the basin.

Fill the bottle again. Take a *very deep* breath and blow out again. Compare your normal breathing with your full lung capacity.

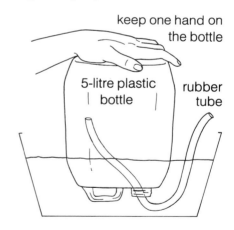

keep one hand on the bottle

5-litre plastic bottle

rubber tube

Questions

1 **Describe how food is prevented from getting into the windpipe.**
2 **How are the air passages swept clean? What damages this process?**
3 **Explain how vigorous exercise can increase your lung capacity.**
4 **What are the usual reasons for food 'going down the wrong way'? Describe how you would help a friend who was choking.**
5 **You are minding a 7-year-old who breathes through his open mouth. It is a bitterly cold, blustery day. Discuss how you would explain to the child that it is healthier to breathe through the nose than the mouth.**

Facts about blood (1)

Blood looks dramatic – grown men have been known to faint at the sight of it! We talk of 'life's blood', 'blood and guts', 'blood freezing in our veins'. Blood is pumped from the heart (p. 94) to carry vital things such as oxygen, food, and hormones to your body, and to take away waste. It also helps fight infection (p. 18), and heals wounds. A man has between 5 and 6 litres of blood; a woman has about a litre less.

The red blood cells

Inside blood are millions of tiny red cells – about 5½ million in each cubic millimetre of blood! Red cells do a vital job: they pick up oxygen from the lungs and transport it round your body. They only last about four months and then have to be replaced. Two million red cells are destroyed and replaced *every second* in your body.

Iron is needed to make healthy red cells. Foods rich in iron are liver, beef, eggs, and pulses. During the teens, and all your life, you must make sure you have enough of these foods in your diet. The growth spurt and the other body changes which happen can run down your store of iron.

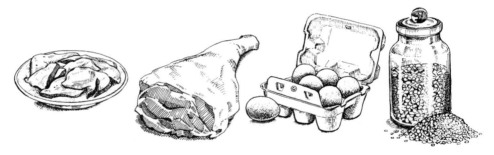

Anaemia

Your body cells use oxygen to 'burn up' food. This sets free the energy you need to live a healthy, active life. If something goes wrong with the red blood cells, less oxygen gets to your body cells and you lack energy. The symptoms of **anaemia** are pale skin, weakness, fainting, and feeling tired *all the time*. It is a condition only a doctor should diagnose (decide). Blood is taken from the arm and sent to a laboratory for examination and a red cell count. Injections of iron or iron tablets are given.

1 Women need more iron in their diet than men because of the blood loss during their periods.
2 A few women become slightly anaemic if they have *very* heavy periods.
3 Pregnant and breast-feeding mothers need more iron in their diet.
4 There is a risk of slight anaemia in the early teens, and girls between 15 and 18 need extra iron in their diet.

Black Americans and Africans may suffer from **Sickle-Cell Anaemia**. This is an inherited weakness of the red cells. People from Mediterranean countries may have a similar condition. These are serious anaemias and pregnant women need very special care, as do their newly-born babies.

Fainting

A faint is a brief loss of consciousness – you 'pass out' and fall down. It is caused by not enough blood being pumped up to the brain. Once the head is lower than the heart, blood flows to the brain and you quickly 'come round'. Two or three faints in a year are not at all serious. More, and you should see a doctor. Care should be taken to avoid faints.

1 Elderly people may faint if they rise quickly after stooping or lying down.
2 Getting out of bed after a long illness can cause faintness. Move slowly.
3 Very hot baths should be avoided. So should spinning round too quickly.
4 Standing still in strong sunlight or hot stuffy rooms causes faintness – think of soldiers on parade and school assembly halls.
5 Do you faint at the sight of blood? An emotional shock can also cause a faint.

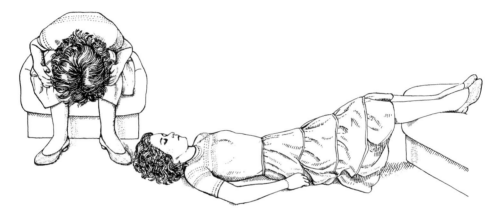

People usually feel weak and unsteady just before they faint. Can you work out why they should lie down with their feet up, or put their head between their knees? It is not good for the brain to be short of oxygen, even for the brief time a faint lasts. Also, there is a risk of other injuries when you fall.

First aid

If someone faints, either shade the person from the sun, or open the windows and doors wide. Loosen any tight clothing around the neck and waist. Raise the feet so they are above the head. The blood will then flow more quickly to the brain. Encourage the person to lie still for a while. Give sips of cool water, then help the person to rise – very slowly.

Questions

1 **How much blood does (a) the average man and (b) the average woman have?**
2 **What foods are rich in iron? Explain the importance of iron in diet.**
3 **Copy out the four points listed under 'Anaemia'.**
4 **What are the symptoms of anaemia, and how is it diagnosed?**
5 **What causes fainting? Why should people take care to avoid faints?**
6 **Choose a partner and role play first aid for a faint.**

Facts about blood (2)

How a cut heals

When you cut yourself, three things must happen quickly:

1 Germs inside the wound must be destroyed (p. 18).
2 Other germs must be prevented from getting into the wound.
3 The bleeding must be stopped.

Your body defences make a **blood clot**. Tiny thread-like strands form in the wound. The strands harden into a plug which stops the bleeding. No more germs can get in as the hardened plug becomes a scab. Under the scab, a new layer of skin is being formed. When this is ready, the scab drops off naturally. Foods rich in Vitamin K, such as dark green leafy vegetables, help blood to clot.

Thrombosis

Not all blood clots are caused by cuts on the surface. The tubes which carry blood may become roughened and damaged on their inside walls. If a blood clot forms, it can block the tube. This is called a **thrombosis**. It is very dangerous. When blood cannot travel to a part of the body, that part will die from lack of oxygen.

A thrombosis in the brain lowers the amount of oxygen taken to the brain cells. This happens in a **stroke**, which can stop a large part of the brain working, or cause death. How strokes are best avoided is discussed on pp. 94–5, which deal with the health of the heart.

Haemophilia

A few males inherit a condition called **haemophilia**. Their blood does not clot properly. When they cut themselves, even slightly, they bleed a great deal. Can you imagine how this is likely to affect their lives? Treatment is by taking clotting factors from stored blood.

Blood doning

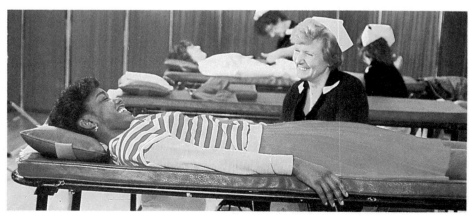

Not everyone's blood group is the same. There are four main groups: A, B, AB, and O. Everyone belongs to one of these groups. A person who gives blood to a **bloodbank** is called a **donor**. You can start giving blood regularly at 18, providing you are in good health and not taking certain medicines. Blood doning is quick and simple. About 500 ml (two small cupfuls) are taken from a vein in your arm. The blood is marked with your blood group and stored in the hospital's bloodbank. Blood doning does not hurt, though you may feel a slight sting as the needle goes in. You rest for a short while afterwards, and then go on your way. It can be very satisfying to think about the stranger who is now fit and healthy thanks to the anonymous gift of your blood. Blood doning is important social work. Will you give blood?

Antibodies

Some germs have such strong poisons that they cannot be destroyed by the white blood cells. Your body defences make chemicals which are called **antibodies** to fight these germs. You do not make antibodies until you have been in contact with the disease. For every different type of germ a matching antibody has to be made. Antibodies stay in the blood to protect you from catching the disease again. This is called having an **immunity**. You are only immune against the diseases you have made antibodies for. These are likely to be such childhood diseases as chicken-pox and mumps. Your body defences cannot make antibodies against all germs. Have you caught a cold more than once in your life?

Immunization

Some childhood diseases are so dangerous it is better to be **immunized** against them first. A solution of very, very weak or dead germs is given. Without catching the disease, the body is tricked into making antibodies. This is artificial immunization. Children are immunized against a number of diseases (pp. 150–1). If you travel to foreign countries, you will need immunizations against the different diseases you might be in contact with.

Finding out:
Immunizations for foreign travel.

Choose a country with a climate very different to yours. Visit your local travel agency and ask which immunizations you will need and what diseases they will protect you from.

r = Vaccinations or tablets recommended for protection against disease

Country	Cholera	Malaria	Typhoid	Polio	Yellow Fever
Kiribati			r	r	
Korea (North)	r		r	r	
Korea (South)	r	r	r	r	
Kuwait	r		r	r	
Laos (Lao)	r	r	r	r	
Lebanon	r		r	r	
Lesotho	r		r	r	

Questions

1 **When you cut yourself, what three things must happen, and why?**
2 **Give a 10-year-old child all the reasons why a scab should not be picked.**
3 **Blood clots are not always helpful. Explain where and how they can be very dangerous indeed.**
4 **What is meant by 'haemophilia'?**
5 **Write a short essay, describing blood doning.**

Teeth and gums

Look at your teeth in a mirror. Count them. An adult has 32 permanent teeth. Your wisdom or back teeth appear between the ages of 17 and 21. Examine your gums for sore red places which may mean **gum disease**. Pass your tongue over your teeth to feel for slightly rough sticky patches. This is **plaque**, a mixture of mucus, food particles, and bacteria germs.

Enamel is very hard for biting and for protecting the tooth.
Dentine is heavy like bone to help grind the food down.
Pulp is soft, with blood tubes and nerves for heat, cold, pressure, and pain.
Roots and **cement** hold the tooth firmly in the jaw.

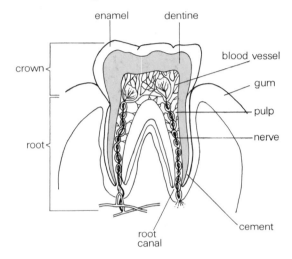

Dental decay

The bacteria in plaque break down the sugar in food, and acid is formed. Acid eats into the enamel and a tiny **cavity** (hole) is made. If this is not filled, the bacteria pass through the dentine and start to breed in the pulp. White blood cells try to fight the infection and the pulp becomes swollen, causing toothache. If the decay is still not treated, the tooth will die.

Visits to the dentist

You can see that an early visit to the dentist stops decay getting past the enamel. If you only go to the dentist when you have toothache, a great deal of damage has already been done. Some people put off going for the six monthly check-up because they don't like pain. This doesn't make sense. Can you work out why?

Gum disease

Gingivitis is the medical name for sore gums which bleed when you clean your teeth. It is caused by the bacteria in plaque spreading to the gums. If gingivitis isn't treated, pockets of pus form around the roots of the teeth. In time, the roots wither, the gums shrink back and the tooth falls out. Two out of three people between the ages of 16 and 35 have some gum disease.

It is sad to lose teeth. **Dentures** (false teeth) have to be fitted and they can be uncomfortable. Because there are no roots left to hold the jaw nice and firm, the lower half of the face looks drawn in and puckered.

Have you an attractive smile?

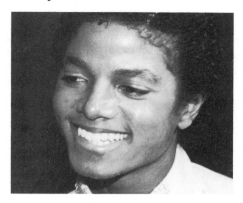

Slightly crooked teeth do not matter – they add interest to your smile. But if your teeth do need straightening, go to the dentist *now* before your wisdom teeth come through. A strong brace will slowly push or pull them back into shape. A broken tooth or rough edge may damage the skin of your mouth or tongue. It needs to be filed smooth, or capped with an artificial crown.

Early tooth care

Milk teeth start to grow in the gums before birth. The first of the twenty appear between 6 and 7 months. Milk teeth must be cared for from the beginning so that the permanent teeth grow down in the right place. Pregnant women and children need a diet rich in calcium foods, proteins, and Vitamins A, C, and D. Parents should train children in proper dental care.

Your dental care

1 Brush teeth up and down after meals and last thing at night. Clean between crowded teeth with dental floss.
2 Use a fluoride toothpaste as it helps protect teeth against decay.
3 Rinse with water, forcing it between teeth. At school or work, finish a meal with a raw vegetable – chewing keeps roots and gums healthy.
4 Cut down on sweet and sticky foods.
5 Do not use your teeth to open things.

Finding out:
If there is plaque on your teeth.

A disclosing tablet has a dye which stains plaque. Chew a tablet to colour any plaque. Remove the stains with floss and a toothbrush. How long does it take you to clean your teeth thoroughly?

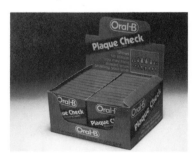

Questions

1 **How many permanent teeth are there? How many milk teeth?**
2 **What is plaque? How is it removed?**
3 **What things happen *before* a tooth begins to ache?**
4 **Explain why people should go for a check-up every six months.**
5 **What is gingivitis? What happens if it is not treated?**
6 **Copy the drawing of a typical tooth. Write down the function of each part.**

Nutrition (1)

The food we eat can affect our health in many ways, so it is very important to know which foods to choose and why. **Nutrients** are the substances in food which provide energy and the raw materials for healthy growth and cell repair. Proteins, carbohydrates, fats, vitamins, and minerals are all nutrients. Most foods contain more than one kind of nutrient. Human milk has all the nutrients a baby needs in the first months of life.

Proteins

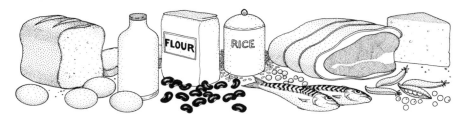

These are essential for growth and body-building, and for replacing worn-out cells and repairing damaged ones. They are especially important for women who are pregnant or breast-feeding; for babies, children, and adolescents who are all growing; and for people who are recovering from an illness or injury. Proteins can also be used to provide energy if the diet lacks enough energy-giving foods.

Animal foods which are good sources of protein include fish, chicken, liver, and meat. Protein foods from animal products include cheese, eggs, and milk. Proteins from plants are found in bread, rice, nuts, beans, and lentils. Plant proteins are an important part of the diet as they are also a good source of energy-giving nutrients.

Carbohydrates

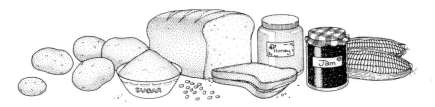

These are the energy-giving foods. Energy is needed all the time. Even while we are asleep, food must be burned with oxygen to provide energy for the lungs to breathe, the heart to pump, and so on. Very active people needs lots of carbohydrates to replace the energy they use up. If more is eaten than the body needs, the excess is turned into fat.

Good sources of carbohydrate are starches (e.g. bread, potatoes, rice) and sugars (e.g. sweets, jams). Starchy foods are the healthy way to get energy because they contain other important nutrients too. Sugar supplies only energy, which is stored as fat if it is not used up. People would be healthier if they cut right down on sugar and sugary foods. They are very fattening. Being obese (very overweight) can lead to heart disease (p. 94) and other serious illnesses. Being obese also tends to make people unhappy, which can lead to stress (p. 71). Sugar also causes tooth decay (p. 40).

Fats

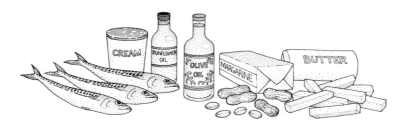

Fats and oils supply energy too. They also make up the body's main store of food. Fats such as margarine and butter also supply other nutrients, including vitamins A, D, and K. Fats also help to keep the body warm. But fats are very fattening — they provide twice the energy value of carbohydrates.

Animal fats are found in butter, cheese, meat, sardines, and eggs. Vegetable oils from plants include margarine, peanuts, and cooking oils. Most animal fats are 'saturated' with the chemical **cholesterol**, which is useful in small amounts in the body. Many vegetable oils are not: they are therefore called 'polyunsaturated'. Too much cholesterol in the blood can cause damage and lead to heart disease (p. 94). It is best to cut down the amount of fat we eat altogether, and to eat vegetable oils rather than animal fats.

Dietary goals

In industrialized countries, poor eating habits can lead to ill health. Heart disease (p. 94), anaemia (p. 36), and tooth decay (p. 40) are a few examples. Dietary goals are set to help people eat *enough* of the *right kinds* of nutrients — and not too much of the wrong kinds. Today's main dietary goals include:

1 Breast milk for babies.
2 Eating less sugar and sugary foods.
3 Eating less fat, especially animal fat.
4 Having far more fibre in the diet (p. 45).

Questions

1 **What are nutrients?**
2 **Why are proteins important? Name three groups of people with special needs for protein.**
3 **What are carbohydrate foods? How can sugar be damaging to health?**
4 **Name three foods rich in animal fats. Briefly explain why people should eat only very small amounts of these.**
5 **What is meant by 'dietary goals'? Copy out today's goals.**
6 **Describe your favourite meal. Then list any foods in it which might cause health problems.**

Nutrition (2)

Vitamins and minerals

These are called **micro-nutrients**. The body needs tiny amounts of them. Vitamins and minerals are found in a wide variety of foods and most people have plenty if they eat a varied diet. Often they work *together* with other nutrients – for example, bones and teeth need proteins, calcium, and vitamin D to grow healthy and strong.

The main vitamins and minerals needed

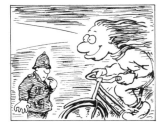

Vitamin A for night vision.

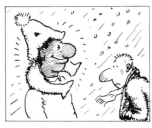

Vitamins A and C to guard against colds and infections.

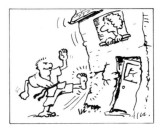

Vitamin D and calcium for strong bones.

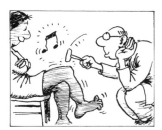

Calcium, sodium, and the Vitamin B group for muscle tone.

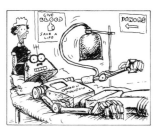

Vitamin B_{12} for replacing blood cells.
Iron for healthy red blood cells.
Salt for blood liquids.
Vitamin K to help blood clot.

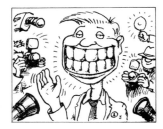

Vitamin C for healthy gums.
Fluoride to protect against tooth decay.
Calcium for healthy teeth.

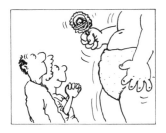

Iodine salts for proper growth.

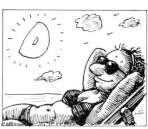

Vitamins C and A for healthy skin.
Vitamin D can be made in sunlight by the skin.

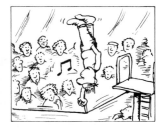

Sodium chloride (salt), calcium, and the Vitamin B group for nerves.

Vitamins in the body	
Vitamins	*Best foods*
A (can be stored in the liver)	Fish-liver oils, sardines, liver, carrots, apricots, spinach, milk and butter, fresh green vegetables
B_1 (cannot be stored)	Yeast, wheat germ, egg yolk, liver, soya beans
B_2 and other B vitamins	Yeast, milk, cheese, kidneys, peanuts, meat, poultry
C (lost by over-cooking or storing)	Citrus fruits, tomatoes, onions, pineapples, berries, green vegetables
D (can be made in skin in sunlight and stored)	Fish-liver oils, eggs, liver, milk
K (stored in liver)	Dark-green leafy vegetables – also found in most foods

Dietary fibre

Fibre makes up the cell walls of plant foods – cereals, vegetables, and fruit. Although it is not digested, fibre is a very important part of our diet. Because it is bulky and absorbent, it helps the muscles of the intestine to push waste food out of the body easily. This prevents constipation (p. 49) and other disorders related to it.

Many foods we eat are 'refined', which means that most of the fibre has been removed. Foods rich in fibre include bran, wholemeal flour and bread, peas and beans, and the skins of fruit and baked potatoes.

Water

Water is essential for life. It is used in the blood for carrying food and oxygen to the cells, and for taking away waste. It helps with the chemical changes in the cells, and keeps the body temperature even. Almost three-quarters of the body weight is water. The average adult loses four to six pints each day by sweating, by passing urine, and by breathing out. (Have you noticed how your breath will steam up a spoon?) All this lost water must be replaced each day.

Questions

1 **What are micro-nutrients? Name two which work together.**
2 **'Night vision' means being able to see in dim light. Which vitamin helps? Name three foods it is found in.**
3 **Name two vitamins which help you have clear skin, glossy hair, and sparkling eyes.**
4 **What importance does fluoride have in the body?**
5 **Name one nutrient and two micro-nutrients needed for healthy bones and teeth.**
6 **What is dietary fibre? Why is it important?**
7 **How much water is lost each day? Why is it essential that this water is replaced? Give as many reasons as you can.**

How much food do you need?

If the amount of food you eat each day equals the amount of energy you use, then you stay in a steady state. But if you eat less or more, then you lose or gain weight. The amount of energy you use depends on your age, your sex, the type of work you do, the climate you live in, how much exercise you take, and – most important – the rate at which food is 'burned' in the cells. This is very different from person to person.

How much food is enough?

Energy is measured in units called **Calories**. The metric unit is the **kilojoule** and one Calorie is equal to 4.2 kilojoules. Men need 2,800 Calories a day; women need 2,300. Athletes and manual workers need about 4,000 Calories. But Calories, like weight charts, have little meaning in the teens as you are still developing. You have to rely on how fit you feel. Whether you are skinny or curvy, if you feel fit and active you are eating the right amounts. But if your size bothers you *and you don't feel fit*, you need to adjust your eating habits.

Approximate number of Calories needed each day:

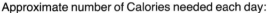

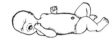

0-6 months
500-720 C

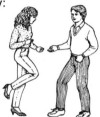

Adolescents:
male 2880 C
female 2300 C

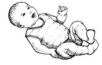

6-12 months
810-980 C

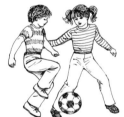

Active children
2000 C

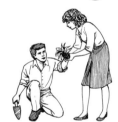

Adults:
male 2800 C
female 2300 C

Adjusting eating habits

Wrong eating habits can be changed, but you have to be strict with yourself. They come from the way you feel about food, so your intelligence has to be trained to take charge of these feelings (pp. 64–5). Your stomach also has to be trained to expect different amounts of food. Both these trainings take a long time. Do not expect rapid results. Remember that exercise is important to help muscles and bones adjust to your new shape.

Eating too little?

Foods rich in vegetable fats and starches are good for weight gain. You also need high protein foods and the micro-nutrients too. Try to drink at least 1 pint of milk each day – add flavourings if you dislike the taste. Concentrate on foods you really enjoy but make sure you have a varied diet. *Eat more of everything.*

Anorexia

This is a behaviour disorder (p. 107) that happens to a few teenagers, usually girls. They stop eating, or they eat and then get rid of the food by vomiting or using laxatives (p. 49). Anorexia can be triggered off by upset feelings over the fashion to be slim, or by hidden worries about growing up. Anorexia is a serious and sad disorder. The girl looks gaunt, her skin dries and ages, body hair may grow and head hair fall out. Her periods stop and her whole development slows down. A few girls have actually starved themselves to death. Treatment is by psychotherapy (p. 91) but it does not always work. Never go on a 'crash' or 'starvation' diet as there is a slight risk of becoming anorexic.

Eating too much?

If you eat more food than you use, the rest is stored as fat. Even though you may eat less than other people, you are still eating too much for you. Cut out fried foods and sugary foods. Concentrate on watery, fibrous, low-fat, low-carbohydrate foods such as salads. *Eat less of everything*. Be strict but not cruel with yourself. Eat a little less each day. Do it *very slowly*, or you will start eating more again.

Self help

1 Milk is nearly the perfect food. Drink at least a pint each day.
2 Too much coffee or tea is not good for you. Drink fruit juice instead.
3 Drink water after exercise and whenever you are thirsty – at least three pints each day.
4 Check how much sugary food you eat. Having a 'sweet tooth' is habit; you can change it by slow training. Eat a little less sugary food each day.
5 Stay away from animal fats. Instead of frying foods, grill sausages, boil potatoes, poach eggs.
6 Hungry teenagers need lots of protein and carbohydrate foods (not sugars). Be proud of your appetite.
7 Check your diet for iron. If you dislike liver, eat beef or wholemeal bread instead.
8 Check your diet for body-building foods – proteins, calcium, vitamin D.
9 If you keep catching colds, increase your intake of vitamin C and A foods.
10 Light-skinned people make their own vitamin D in sunshine. Dark-skinned people need to make sure they have plenty of vitamin D in their diet.

Questions

1 **Write a short essay, explaining clearly why it is important that the amount of food you eat should equal the amount of energy you use.**
2 **What is a Calorie? How many Calories do men, women, and athletes need each day? Convert these figures into kilojoules.**
3 **How can you best judge the amount of food you need?**
4 **Name three foods which are good for weight gain and say why.**
5 **Write a short account of the proper way to lose weight.**
6 **Plan a meal for a hungry teenager. List the nutrients in each type of food you include.**

About food in the body

Before food can be used, it has to be broken down into simpler things. This is called **digestion**, and it happens in the **food canal**. Proteins are broken down into amino-acids, carbohydrates into simple sugars, and fats into glycerol and fatty acids. They pass into the blood and are taken to the cells. Here they 'burn' with oxygen and energy is released for all the body's work. Micro-nutrients, alcohol, and many drugs can pass straight into the blood.

The food canal

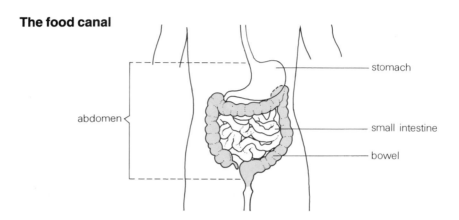

Most digestion happens in the **stomach** and the **small intestine** (guts). The small intestine is, in fact, over six metres long! But it is much narrower than the last part, the **bowel**, which deals with waste. Both the bowel and the small intestine lie, coiled and looped, in the **abdomen**. The abdomen is that large area below the ribs often called the 'belly' or 'tummy'.

Food hygiene

Germs get into the food canal when you eat infected food – this is called food poisoning. Foods can be infected before you buy them, or while they are being prepared at home. Check your personal hygiene. Always wash your hands in hot soapy water before preparing food and after using the toilet. Be scrupulously clean in the kitchen: no sneezing, no dirty handkerchiefs, no loose, hanging hair.

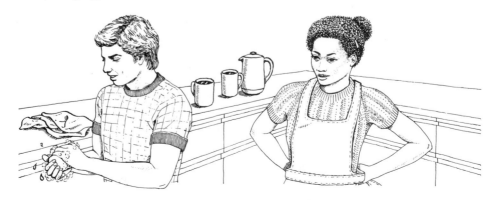

Diarrhoea

Infected food may be vomited from the stomach quite soon after it is eaten. More usually, the germs are busy breeding in the food canal before you begin to feel ill. White blood cells rush to destroy them, and the liquid food is hurried through the large intestine and out of the bowel. You can see why diarrhoea is often called 'the runs'.

Diarrhoea stops when the infection clears up. During the attack, a great deal of water and important micro-nutrients may be lost. It is a serious disease in babies as they quickly become dehydrated (dried out) and ill. The lost water must be replaced and the baby taken to a doctor if the diarrhoea lasts more than a day. Extra hygiene is very important, or the infection will spread to other people in the house.

Constipation

Part of the food you eat, including dietary fibre, cannot be broken down. It travels to the bowel where it forms into **faeces** (stools). Bowel movements are the passing of faeces out of the body by powerful muscles. People have very different bowel movements: four times a day, once a day, once every four days – or anything in between.

If faeces are not passed regularly, they become thick, hard, and dry. They are uncomfortable to pass. Constipation is quite common in the teens as many adolescents do not drink enough water. **Laxatives** are medicines to soften the faeces – they should be avoided. There is a risk they might cause the powerful muscles of the bowel to lose their muscle tone (p. 30).

Self help

1 Constipation is not serious. If you worry, you make it worse.
2 Go to the toilet at the same time each day *and* when you have plenty of time.
3 If nothing happens after ten minutes, don't worry. Try again the next day.
4 Drink up to six pints of water a day. You will find it really works.
5 Make sure you have enough dietary fibre (p. 45). It improves bowel muscle tone and keeps the faeces bulky and soft.
6 Have plenty of exercise. There is no better way to improve muscle tone.

Questions

1 **What is meant by 'digestion', and where does it happen?**
2 **Name the three nutrients which are broken down, and say into what.**
3 **Where does most digestion happen?**
4 **What is the function of the bowel?**
5 **What causes diarrhoea? Why is it often called 'the runs'?**
6 **In its normal healthy state, the bowel is full of germs. Write a short essay on the importance of hygiene, when using the toilet, and before preparing food.**
7 **What are laxatives? Why should they be avoided?**

Your eyes and their care

Many people think that sight is the most important of the senses. Do you agree? List at least ten things you would not be able to do if you were blind.

How your eye is protected

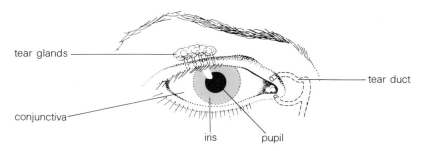

Eyebrows stop sweat and rain running into your eyes. Eyelids work as shutters, closing down to let your eyes rest. They also blink quickly if anything comes too close (p. 63). Eyelashes work as traps, stopping bits of dust and grime from entering the eye. The **conjunctiva** is a transparent lining which covers the eyeball *and* the inside of the eyelid.

From the diagram, notice where the tear glands are. Tears are slightly salty and slightly antiseptic. They are made all the time. Blinking spreads the tear across the eye, keeping it clean and damp. The tear ducts at the inside corner drain the fluid into the back of the nose. Study the structure of your eye using a magnifying glass and a mirror.

How light enters the eye

The **pupil** is the dark hole in the middle of the eye. It is surrounded by rings of coloured muscle, the **iris**. Light rays pass through the pupil and land on sensitive light cells, the **retina**, at the back of the eye. Too much light is damaging, so the iris closes up, letting in only a small amount of light. When the light is dim, the iris opens wide to let in all the light there is.

The work of the lens

Behind each pupil is a **lens**, which is transparent to let light through. The lens is held in place by muscles and ligaments. When you look at distant objects, the lens is flat and thin. When you do close work, such as reading, the muscles pull the lens, making it short and fat. This is because the lens has the power to **refract** (bend) light, so that a clear, sharp image lands on the retina.

Long and short sight

People who are born long-sighted cannot see close objects clearly. The lens doesn't become short and fat enough to bend the light to make a sharp image on the retina. Spectacles (glasses) which bend the light more will correct this condition.

People who are born short-sighted cannot see distant objects clearly. The lens doesn't become long and thin enough to focus the light on the retina. Again, spectacles with specially-made lenses will correct this.

As people get older, the muscles which pull the lens may become slightly weaker. Many people over forty need spectacles for reading and close work.

Eye infections

A **stye** is an infection caused by germs in the tiny oil glands along the eyelid. The lump may be small, but it feels very painful. Bathe it regularly with clean cotton wool soaked in warm water. If you keep getting styes, go to your doctor for a general check-up on your health.

Conjunctivitis is an infection of the conjunctiva. It is sometimes called 'pink-eye' as the transparent lining turns pink and sore. Conjunctivitis is very contagious (catching). Be careful not to use other people's towels or flannels, and to wash your hands if you touch your eyes. Go to the doctor if this infection does not clear up in a few days.

Self help
1 Your eyes and sight are precious and need to be looked after. Regular check-ups are important. If you need spectacles, *wear* them.
2 Vitamin A foods – liver, eggs, green vegetables – keep your eyes healthy.
3 Make sure you have a good light directed *on* your work when you study.
4 Rest your eyes now and then by staring into the distance during study.
5 Always wear protective goggles if there are splinters flying around.
6 When grit gets in the eye, tears pour down to wash it out. If this doesn't work, pull the eyelid gently back and remove it with a clean tissue.

Finding out:
How the iris works.

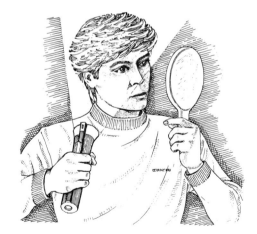

Sit in a dark room with a torch in front of a mirror. Shine the torch into your eyes and you will see the iris starting to close.

Questions

1 **Explain how your eye is protected from dust and grime.**
2 **Write a short account of how the iris controls the amount of light entering the eye.**
3 **What is the lens? Explain its work.**
4 **Write about two infections which can occur to the eye.**
5 **Copy out the self-help points. Try to learn them.**

Any aches and pains?

Aches and pains

These are symptoms (signs) that something is going wrong. Everyone gets them from time to time. Often it's easy to work out why. Stuffy rooms, loud music, or late nights can give you a headache; over-exercise or swimming after a meal will give you cramp. Aches and pains are your body's way of protesting at the treatment it is getting.

Reaching for the tablets

In a few homes, as soon as a headache begins, aspirins are taken; at the slightest sore throat, syrupy linctus is swallowed. But medicines you buy from the chemist ease the aches and pains for a while only. The trouble will start up again as soon as the effects have worn off.

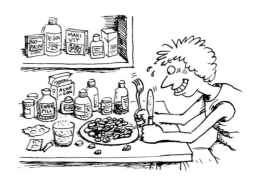

What to do?

Stop mistreating yourself! Your body has its own in-built recovery system which works perfectly, if you let it. Once you have stopped whatever caused the aches and pains, check your diet and the amount of sleep, fresh air, and exercise you are getting. Then wait, and you will find you are fit and healthy again.

Pain

Pain is a curious thing. It is felt in the *mind*, not at the place where you hurt. Some people are more sensitive to pain than others. This does not mean they are less brave. And there are different ways of reacting to pain too, depending on the person's state of mind. For example, an athlete in a thrilling race accepts the pain of over-exertion, yet may cringe away from the tiny prick of the needle when giving blood. Think of pain as a warning, and a protection against further damage. What might happen if there was no such thing as pain?

When to go to the doctor

1 **Persistent pain** This kind doesn't stop. It may be quite mild, but it becomes unbearable because your resistance to it gets lower and lower.
2 **Regular pain** This can come and go at fairly regular times. After meals, at night or in the early morning – it is likely to recur at the same time each day.
3 **Moving pain** This can come and go in different places at different times. It may be caused by hidden worries, or there may be something physically wrong. Either way, you do need to talk it over with your doctor.

Doctors

Doctors are people. Some are better than others. But on average they are very good, perhaps because of their long training. Don't be put off if your doctor seems rushed. This is not unusual, and you will get the help you need. Home visits are only made if you are far too ill to get to the surgery. Telephone before ten o'clock for an appointment.

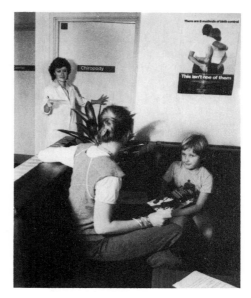

Some doctors have **group practices**. They work together from the same surgery. If you feel happier with one particular doctor, ask for your doctor by name when you telephone for an appointment. Other doctors hold their surgeries in **community health centres**. These provide a wide range of medical services, such as immunization, dental care, and treatment for the elderly, all under one roof.

Communication

Doctors are not mind-readers. They cannot guess what is wrong with you. Try not to mumble from shyness or embarrassment. Decide exactly what to say before you leave home. Explain your symptoms clearly and describe the pain – is it dull, sharp, or throbbing? Point to the trouble spot if you don't know its name. Then listen very carefully. A recent study found that many patients do not listen to their doctor's instructions. If you don't understand something, ask the doctor to explain it, and then follow the instructions for treatment exactly.

Self help

1 Your body has its own in-built recovery system. The best self help usually means waiting for things to settle down.
2 If your pain is at all worrying, you should see the doctor.
3 Try not to be embarrassed. Doctors have heard it all many times before.
4 Don't be disappointed if you are not given a prescription (p. 54). If may be advice you need, rather than treatment.

Questions

1 **What is meant by a 'symptom'? Name two symptoms of the common cold.**
2 **Give two reasons why you might have a headache.**
3 **When should you visit the doctor? Name the three kinds of pain.**
4 **Copy out the self-help points into your book.**
5 **Choose a partner and role play (a) making an appointment by telephone and (b) describing the symptoms of your headache to the doctor.**

Facts about drugs

Drugs are medicines used to cure illness, deaden pain, prevent the spread of disease, and maintain health. Drugs have been used for thousands of years. They come from chemicals in the roots, leaves, seeds, bark, and juices of plants. A few come from animals, and some are artificially made in laboratories. **Antibiotics** are drugs which can kill **bacteria**, the larger germs. They cannot kill **viruses**, which are smaller. This is why people with viral infections are not always given drugs.

Digitalis comes from the foxglove and is used for heart disease.

Side effects

Drugs speed up, block off, or otherwise interfere with the body's work. They need to be able to do this without causing too many **side effects** (other kinds of damage). Antibiotics must not kill off healthy cells. Drugs for skin disorders should not scar. **Narcotics** (drugs for deadening great pain) should not damage the other senses. All this is very difficult indeed.

The safe dose

Because they interfere with the body, drugs are bound to have some side effects. Usually they are minor things like diarrhoea or constipation; feeling giddy, faint, or sick. A safe dose is worked out for each different patient: things like height, weight, age, sex, and past illness are taken into account. A safe dose will have the least side effects for that particular person. A safe dose is not 'safe' for anyone else.

At the chemist's

Drugs from the chemist are sold under their trade names – which is why they are called **patent medicines**. Usually they do not cure, but they can soothe aches and pains. Always ask the chemist's advice before buying. Read the instructions before leaving the shop. Make sure you know how to take the drug, and whether there are any side effects.

Drug control

A drug which is controlled can only be prescribed by a doctor. These include the powerful antibiotics and narcotics. A **prescription** is the written direction for a controlled drug to be made up. Any other way of obtaining these drugs is illegal, and drug-smuggling is a serious crime (p. 107). As well as protecting people from drug abuse, there are important medical reasons why powerful drugs are controlled.

1 **Tolerance** This means the body becomes 'used to' the drug. Larger and more frequent doses would be needed. The side effects could cause death.
2 **Allergy** This means the body reacts dangerously to a drug. Penicillin is one drug to which some people are allergic. The person would be very ill indeed, without knowing why.
3 **Resistance** Bacteria can build up resistance to certain drugs. If they were used too often, they would become useless for curing disease.
4 **Addiction** This means the person depends upon a drug, either mentally or physically. Apart from the terrible harm this can do, being addicted to anything means losing your freedom of choice.
5 **Side effects** Even uncontrolled drugs, such as aspirin, can have surprisingly harmful side effects in some people. In large doses, aspirin is fatal. In smaller doses it can cause bleeding from the stomach.

Self help
1 Read the instructions carefully and take the exact dose.
2 Do not try to hurry things along by taking an extra one. Remember side effects.
3 Do not under-dose either. Certain drugs have to be taken over a long period of time before you begin to improve.
4 Take drugs exactly as instructed. For example, before or after food; or with a long drink of water.
5 Finish off a course of drugs, even when you feel better. The hardest germs to kill will be the last. They may linger on, then flare up again.
6 Ask the doctor about side effects. Stop taking the drugs if you notice any other side effects. Inform the doctor at once.
7 Lock drugs safely away in the first-aid box. Throw away unused ones. Never leave drugs where children could reach them.

Finding out:
The words used to describe patent medicines.

Either study the advertisements in magazines, or read the labels on bottles and lotions. Are words like 'cure' used? Make a note of which words are used most often. Have a discussion about the 'hidden persuaders'.

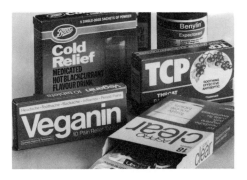

Questions

1 **What are drugs? What things do they come from?**
2 **What is the work of antibiotics? And narcotics?**
3 **In your own words, explain what is meant by a 'safe dose'.**
4 **What are patent medicines? Name any two you know and say what they do.**
5 **Name two controlled drugs. How are they obtained legally?**
6 **Copy out the four medical reasons why drugs are controlled.**
7 **Explain as carefully as you can why people should never 'borrow' or 'lend' medicine prescribed by the doctor.**

Treating a fever

Infectious diseases

1 Germs are *carried to people* by contaminated water and food, by polluted air, by animals – mainly insects and worms.
2 Germs are *passed between people* by direct contact – touching infected persons, or by indirect contact – touching infected things they use.
3 Germs are *spread on one person* by re-infection – picking at spots, scratching at skin infections, unwashed hands after using the toilet.

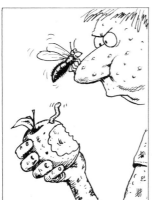 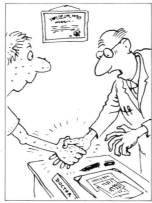 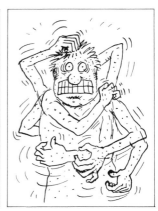

Body temperature

There is no such thing as a 'normal' body temperature. The average is about 36.8° Centigrade, so a few points of degrees above or below is perfectly normal. Body temperature is lowest in the morning and rises slightly during the day. Babies and small children have higher temperatures than adults. Elderly people have lower ones.

Body temperature comes from the heat produced when oxygen 'burns' with food to release energy. Humans have a constant body temperature which allows them to live in very hot or very cold climates. They adapt to different climates by the amount and type of clothes they wear, and the heat in their homes, schools, offices, and so on. In cold countries, special attention must be paid to babies and the elderly. They may suffer **hypothermia** (low body heat) from lack of proper nourishment, exercise, or unheated rooms. But high body temperature is also dangerous. Some babies suffer **hyperthermia** – they are kept far too warm. Cells need a constant body warmth to work efficiently.

Taking a temperature

Body temperature is measured on a Celsius **thermometer**. At first, you may find this difficult to read. Hold the glass end opposite the metal bulb. Turn it very slowly until you see the dark bar of mercury. Notice the Centigrade markings and the tiny arrow showing average body temperature.

Before you begin, check the mercury is down *below* the first marking. If it is above, hold the glass end firmly and give a sharp downwards shake of the wrist. It may need a few shakes before the mercury comes down.

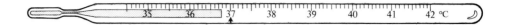

1 Wipe the metal end with cotton-wool dampened with antiseptic.
2 Place the metal end under the tongue. Close the mouth, holding the thermometer with the lips, not the teeth. Do not try to speak.
3 Leave it for a full three minutes before removing it. Read it carefully.
4 Write down the result. Shake down the mercury. Wipe the metal end with antiseptic and return it to its case. Put it away in the first-aid box.

Take a child's temperature under the arm. Tuck the thermometer well in and hold the child's arm across the chest. Never leave a child alone with a thermometer. You will get a falsely high reading if you take a temperature after a hot bath, exercise, or a hot drink.

Fever

The word 'fever' sounds quite alarming but fever itself is *not* a disease. It is the signs of the battle raging between the body's defences and the invading germs. If the germs are very powerful and breeding very rapidly, all the body's energy must be concentrated on destroying them. Other work stops. The battle produces great heat and the body temperature rises.

Other symptoms of fever include: aching all over, shivers of cold then burning heat, intense dryness then heavy sweating, loss of appetite, restlessness, often bad headache. When the temperature is very high, the mind becomes 'feverish', or confused. This is **delirium** and is very rare.

Treating a fever

Go to bed and stay there. The room should be warm, but not hot or stuffy. An electric fan or damp cloths cool the body down. Eat a little if you can, but don't worry about food. You must drink plenty of liquids to replace the water lost by sweating. Aspirin will bring down a temperature and relieve a headache. Telephone for your doctor's advice on this if you are worried. Sleep, doze, rest.

As your temperature drops, read, listen to the radio, or watch television. You will feel more cheerful tucked up on a sofa with a blanket. Try to eat. Go back to bed for short naps. It is quite usual to feel a bit 'low' after a feverish illness – keep your mind occupied.

Questions

1 **Copy out the three main ways in which germs can infect the body.**
2 **What is the average body temperature and how is body heat produced?**
3 **What is hypothermia? What causes it and which groups of people may suffer?**
4 **How is body temperature measured?**
5 **Write a brief description of how you would take a child's temperature.**
6 **Explain why body temperature rises during an infectious disease.**
7 **Name at least four symptoms of a fever.**

Further work on Chapter 1

1   Write a short essay describing the changes which happen in the skin during the teens.

2   Do a project on fashions in hair styles through the ages.

3   Draw or cut out pictures of hair styles you think suitable for today's teenagers. Say why you have chosen these particular styles.

4   Write a full essay, discussing the best ways to resist germs.

5   A younger friend has started getting a few spots. What advice would you give your friend on how to keep acne at bay?

6   Parents of children with head lice are advised to report it to the school. In what ways do you think this is helpful?

7   Test your shoes for correct size. Place each bare foot in turn on a sheet of cardboard and draw around the outline. Cut out the shapes, then slip them into each one of your pairs of shoes. They should lie flat. Do they?

8   Golf, swimming, gymnastics, darts, table-tennis. Say which of these sports may not be vigorous exercise, and why.

9   What are the symptoms of the common cold? How would you help it to clear up?

10 Write a short essay discussing the importance of iron in the diet.

11 Look up the address of the nearest Blood Doning Centre in the telephone book. Write to ask if you may visit them and make notes of their work.

12 Write to the Dental Health Council for more information on their work. Do a full project on the importance of tooth and gum care.

13 Collect wrappers and labels from foods rich in animal and plant fats. Make a list of the ones containing polyunsaturated fats.

14 Write to your local Health Education Office for leaflets on dietary fibre. Do a full project on the importance of fibre in the diet.

15 Choose one day, perhaps at the weekend, and keep a record of the numbers of cups or glasses of liquid you drink. Is it enough?

16 Describe three ways in which the germs of food poisoning can be spread in the kitchen.

17 If possible, visit your local Community Health Centre and make notes on the wide range of medical services going on.

18 'Taking any kind of drug makes some people anxious.' Discuss this statement.

19 Explain why you should always finish a course of antibiotics.

20 A friend is in bed with flu (influenza). It is not serious enough to call a doctor. Describe some of the things you would do to nurse your friend back to health.

Chapter 2

About mental health

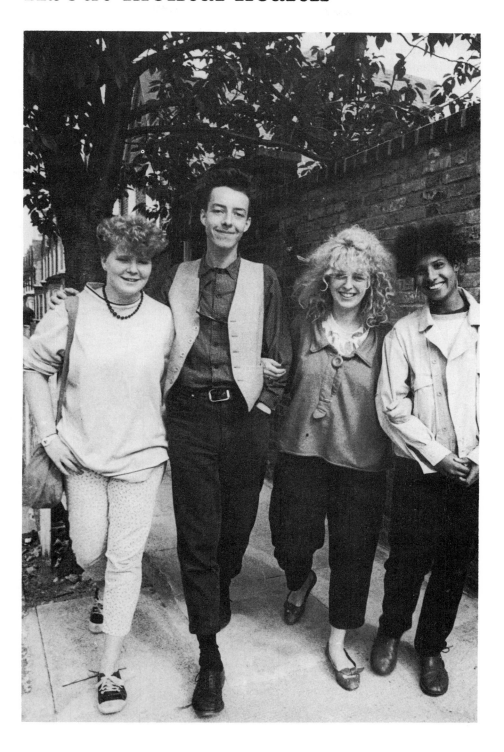

The study of mental health

What is mental health?

Mental health is to do with your mind. It is about the way you think and feel. There are many different definitions of mental health. This is because it is not an easy thing to describe. Perhaps the best definition is the same as for physical health – 'having a sense of well-being'. This will include:

1 Liking yourself and feeling you are a worthwhile person.
2 Feeling good about other people.
3 Being able to face up to the bad as well as the good sides of life.

Imagine you are a person who thinks the opposite of these three points *all the time*. Would you be happy? Would you have a sense of well-being? Notice the words in italics. They are very important. Everyone feels bad about themselves, or other people, or the world *now and then*.

Mental illness

When people lose their sense of well-being *all the time*, they are likely to become mentally ill. One in ten adults will spend a while in a mental hospital. The number of people treated for mental illness at home is increasing at an alarming rate. It is now believed that most mental illness could have been avoided. This chapter is to help you have a better understanding of what goes on inside people's minds.

People are 'different'

Think of a physically healthy person, perhaps yourself or a friend. Do you have freckles or moles? Is one foot slightly larger than the other? These things are not important. They do not mean you are physically ill. But you can see you are 'different'. Everyone is.

It is rather the same with mental health. For example: if you like yourself but sometimes think you don't amount to much, this does not mean you are mentally ill. (You may even get a gloomy kind of pleasure from thinking like this!) The way you feel and think are part of your nature, just as freckles and moles are part of your appearance.

The study of mental health

*'All the world's daft except thee and me,
And I'm not too sure about thee – !''*

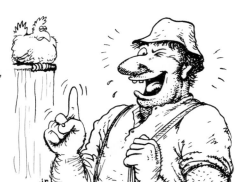

What do you think of this quotation? Does it amuse you, or do you find it boring? You can tell there is no such thing as completely normal behaviour. If there were, people would behave in exactly the same way. Think how boring that would be! Everyone has different areas of light and shade: quirky, interesting, **individual**. The differences between people make human relationships rich and fascinating. It can make them troublesome too. But would you really want everyone to be exactly the same?

In the study of mental health, you must remember people are different. You must respect these differences; not only in others, but in yourself as well.

Comparisons

Because of the physical changes which happen during the teens, people often compare themselves with others to see how they are developing. Sometimes they make **negative** comparisons (judgements against themselves):
'I am not as tall/attractive/popular/witty/clever/good at sport as the others.'
Do you think negative comparisons help people to like themselves and feel worthwhile? Would it be more useful to concentrate on the **positive** ways in which people are different – and to try to respect these differences?

Finding out:
Your best side, or profile.

Hold a sheet of cardboard as in the picture. Study the features of your face, side by side. It is rare to find a face where the right side exactly matches the left. Does yours?

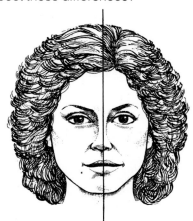

Questions

1 **Give the definition of mental health.**
2 **Copy into your book the three things it includes.**
3 **In the study of mental health, what must you remember?**
4 **Shakespeare wrote: 'Comparisons are odorous.' Do you agree? Give reasons for your answer.**
5 **The 'Finding out' activity is to show there are 'differences' even in your face. Have a discussion on the importance of respecting the differences in people's behaviour.**

What is your 'mind'?

The brain

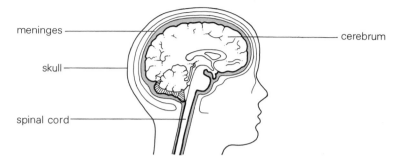

An adult brain weighs about 1.5 kilograms, and is made up of about 15,000 million cells. The **cerebrum** controls your **conscious actions**. These are actions under the control of your will, such as walking and talking. It also deals with things which are not completely understood, such as intelligence, memory, emotion, and imagination. Other parts of the brain control your **unconscious actions**. These are actions you cannot control, such as your heart beat and how much you sweat.

Notice the skull protecting the brain. Feel your own, starting at your eyebrows and going right back over your head. Inside the skull are three linings called the **meninges**. These protect the delicate brain cells and nourish them with oxygen and dissolved foods.

The 'mind'

Your 'mind' is the thinking and feeling part of your brain. But the 'mind' cannot be seen by cutting open a brain. Who can see such things as memory, thoughts, loneliness, or imagination? Nevertheless, although the 'mind' cannot actually be seen, everyone knows what it is.

1 You think with your **intelligence** – the part of your mind which can reason and understand.
2 You feel with your **emotions** – the part of your mind which is 'moved' to sorrow, joy, anger, and so on.

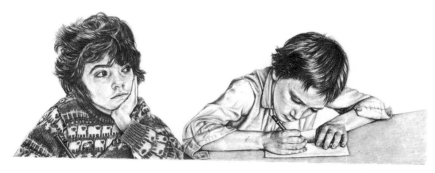

'She's clever, but spends her time day-dreaming.'
'He's not bright, but he'll come first because he works hard.'

Why do these children behave so differently? Which part of the 'mind' do you think each child might be using?

The answers are not important here. What is important is that you understand how people's emotions affect their intelligence – and the other way around. For the purpose of this study, the two things will be discussed as if they are quite separate. Often they are not.

As well as the emotions and the intelligence, one other thing also affects our behaviour. This is *instinct*.

Instinct

If an object suddenly comes too close to your eyes, you blink rapidly. This is a reflex, an instinctive action. It happens without you having to think or feel. Instinctive actions are **inborn**. They do not have to be learned. Instincts are there to protect us, and keep us safe from harm.

But very few of our actions are purely instinctive. For example: babies cry out against loud, sudden noises. But they quickly learn that the noise is Dad banging the front door. This is exciting. Dad plays special games. Instead of crying out, they turn and give Dad big grins.

The psyche

This is pronounced 'sigh-key'. It is the correct word for everything which is meant by the human mind. **Psychology** is the science of how the mind works. **Psychiatry** is the medical treatment for illnesses of the mind. You are not studying psychology or psychiatry. But you need to know these words as they will be used again in this chapter.

Finding out:
If some reflex actions can be controlled.

Blinking protects the eye from getting dusty and dry. People usually blink about once every four seconds. Can you control your blinking for much longer? (Take care not to let your eyes get too dry.)

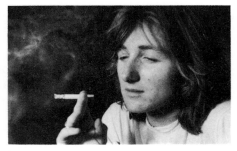

In what way does this show that blinking protects the eyes?

Questions

1 **How much does an adult brain weigh? How many brain cells are there?**
2 **Explain the difference between conscious and unconscious actions.**
3 **What is the function of (a) the skull and (b) the meninges?**
4 **'You think with your ... You feel with your ...' Copy out and learn these two sentences.**
5 **What is the correct word for the human mind? Explain the meanings of (a) psychology and (b) psychiatry.**
6 **Can you control some reflex actions? From what you learned about blinking, is this wise? Give reasons for your answer.**

Facts about intelligence

Intelligence on its own is the power to think, to reason, to know, to understand. Everyone has this power. Some people have more of it than others. But this does not mean they will be happier because they are more intelligent. The most clever people can lead the most miserable lives – and the other way around.

This is because intelligence is *not* one thing on its own. Try to clear your mind of thinking that intelligence is just about doing well at examinations. It is not. Your intelligence is far deeper and wider than this. It includes such things as will-power, self-control, judgement, sensitivity, and stamina (staying power).

Brain development

From before birth, your brain developed earlier than the rest of your body. Have you noticed how a baby's head is large compared with the rest of him?

1 At birth, your brain was 25% of its adult weight.
2 At six months, almost 50%.
3 At two and a half years old, about 75%.
4 By the age of five, nearly 90% of its adult weight.

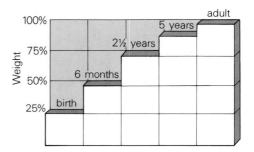

This is an amazing growth spurt. Protein is the growth food (p. 42). You can see why pregnant mothers, babies, and small children must have lots of milk, meat, eggs, fish, and cheese in their diet. Not enough is yet known about brain growth in relation to intelligence, but it is known that a baby learns more in his first two years than in the rest of his life! Also, it is generally agreed that intelligence peaks somewhere between early adolescence and the age of 30. It stays at this level until old age, when there may be a slight decline.

Intelligence and your sex

There is no difference in intelligence among boys and girls. But girls do better on verbal tests – e.g. word fluency, memory work, and reasoning. And boys do better on quantitative (measurements) and spatial (space) tests – e.g. maths and science. It is thought these differences may be a result of upbringing rather than true ability – nobody yet knows.

Intelligence and you

In early adolescence, your intelligence increases. You learn to reason logically; abstract thinking begins. It is thought this increase follows the growth spurt of puberty, which is why girls are ahead of boys till about 14, when boys rapidly catch up. It is thought that you inherit about three-quarters of your intelligence, and the rest comes from your environment. But there is no general agreement on this. The most interesting point is – how much effort do you yourself make?

Will power

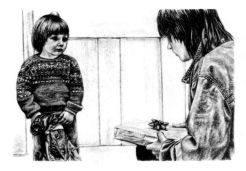

Four-year-old Zack doesn't want to put on his coat. His mother says, 'We don't want to be late for the party. I can't help; I'm carrying the parcel.' Zack's mother appeals to the child's intelligence; his reason (if he goes on fussing they'll be late) and sense of fair play (her hands are full with the parcel). She is teaching Zack to use his will-power to do the things which help him most.

Stamina

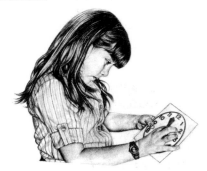

Seven-year-old Zoe is fed up trying to learn to tell the time. Her father says, 'When I was your age, it took me six weeks. You've only been trying for one week.' Zoe's father is teaching Zoe it is necessary to develop staying power in order to learn.

Self help

Both will-power and stamina are important parts of your intelligence. They decide how much effort you yourself make. They are rather like 'mental muscles' – the more you use them, the stronger they become. Whether you think you are bright or not, try to work hard during the teens so that your intelligence peaks at its highest level *for you*.

Questions

1 **Write a short paragraph about early brain development.**
2 **What foods should a baby's diet be rich in, and why?**
3 **Zack's mother could have put the parcel down and forced Zack's arms into his coat. Have a discussion on why she chose to motivate (give him reasons) instead.**
4 **Would Zack need to be motivated to eat an ice cream? Children are motivated by adults to do difficult things. What do you think 'self-motivation' means?**
5 **Zoe hopes to be a gymnast. In what way will her father's teaching help?**
6 **There is a limit to how far body muscles can be trained. This is also true of 'mental muscles'. Explain why you should work hard in the teens whether you are bright or not.**

About the emotions

Self-preservation

Everyone is born with the instinct of self-preservation. This means not only keeping your body safe from harm. It also means keeping your mind in a state of well-being – feeling 'good' about yourself and the world you are in.

Some psychologists believe there are three basic emotions – love, fear and anger. They believe that the other emotions come from these three and are a mixture of them. They also believe that these three emotions grow directly from the instinct of self-preservation, and are very important indeed.

1 **Love** – You love the things which give you pleasure and make you feel safe.
2 **Fear** – You fear the things which make you feel threatened (insecure, unsafe).
3 **Anger** – You are angry when something upsets your pleasure and stops you getting your own way.

Love

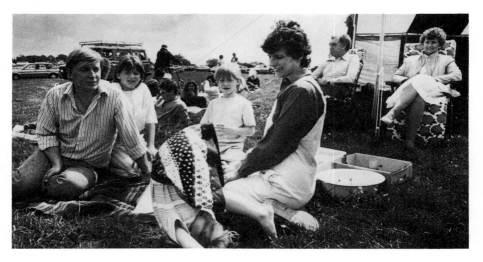

Love is the emotion which makes people happy. And happy people are – on average – healthier than unhappy people. Love could be called the 'health cocktail' as it is a mixture of different ingredients and makes you feel good.

Self love Babies are cuddled, comforted, fed, and kept warm. They feel 'good'. Happy feelings flow to the people who make them feel this way. This is called 'self love' because the baby's love is about *getting* pleasure.

Give-and-take love As the intelligence develops, children understand that to *get* happy feelings they must *give* them too. They try to please their parents. They learn a difficult lesson – to share toys with their friends.

Romantic love At some time in the teens, romantic love becomes a powerful drive. It is so strong it can take you over completely. It can make you blind to the faults of the beloved. Romantic love alone can lead to an unhappy marriage. If it is balanced with the intelligence, it can be the powerful force which helps to make a marriage successful.

Mature love This is a mixture of the other loves, but it is far more outgoing. Emotionally mature adults strive for the happiness of their children, and each other. They look after their friends. They feel responsible for society and do what they can to help others.

Altruistic love This is called the highest form of loving. It means you devote your life to the happiness of others, and do not expect anything in return. Mother Theresa of Calcutta is a fine example of altruistic love. She put high ideals and love of others above herself. She set up fifty schools, orphanages and houses for the poor in India and other countries. She was awarded the Nobel Prize for Peace in 1979.

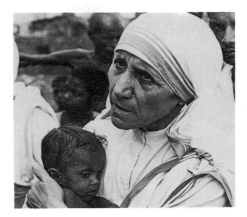

'Love makes the world go round'

If you study the different kinds of love, you will notice that love itself is like the merry-go-round on page 8. People move from one stage of love to the next at more or less the same time as they move from one different stage in life to another. Try to match up these stages.

Self help
Romantic love is bitter-sweet: agony and ecstasy at the same time. A few people spend their teens falling in and out of this bewildering condition! Try not to let romantic love unsteady you too much. Perhaps comfort yourself with the fact that teenage love seldom lasts. This is because neither person yet knows who they really are. It might help to spend a little more time finding out about yourself first.

Finding out:
More about your basic emotions

Make separate lists of things you love, fear, and get angry about. Swop with a friend, or study them on your own. Can you trace some things back to your instinct of self-preservation?

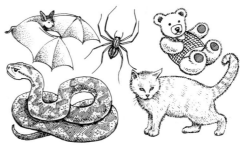

Questions

1 **What is meant by the 'instinct of self-preservation'?**
2 **Copy out the three basic emotions and the sentences beside them.**
3 **In your own words, explain why love is called the 'health cocktail'.**
4 **Find out who was awarded the Nobel Prize for Peace last year, and why. Have a discussion on why love and peace are so often linked together.**
5 **'Love makes the world go round.' Do you agree? Give as many reasons as you can for your answer.**

Fear

Imagine you are alone on a dark night. You hear footsteps behind you, slowly coming near. Your heart thumps loudly, your breath comes in quick gasps. You may turn pale, feel sick, or break out in a cold sweat. Have you noticed how a cat tenses up with fear?

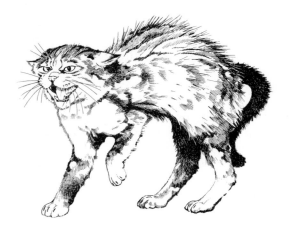

The 'fight or flight' system

Your body reacts automatically to fear. It is instinctive behaviour which you cannot control. **Adrenalin**, sometimes called the 'fear' hormone, pours into your blood. It floods right through your body, speeding up breathing and heart rate. This causes extra oxygen to be rushed to your muscles and an enormous amount of energy is released. Things like digestion and body-building are stopped as they are not important for your immediate survival. Suddenly your whole body has only one interest – to get you out of trouble.

Fight or flight?

Whether you stand and fight or take to your heels in flight depends upon the situation, and the sort of person you are. Whichever you choose, adrenalin has prepared you for action (a) by releasing an enormous amount of energy and (b) by tensing you up. This is very important if your life is actually being threatened. But the more usual fears come from things like being called into the Head's office, or waiting your turn at the dentist. You are tensed up for action, but you know you should not fight or run away. It is likely you must face whatever is going to happen! (See pp. 72–3.)

More about fear

There are many different kinds of fear. Some are serious, others are very mild. Fear can be anything which upsets your sense of safety. Nowadays, it is called 'feeling threatened'. Imagine you are getting ready for the big match, or preparing to go out on an important date – how do you feel? Any sort of challenge can make you feel threatened for a short time.

This sprinter's body is flooded with adrenalin. Can you work out the ways in which it helps him to run faster?

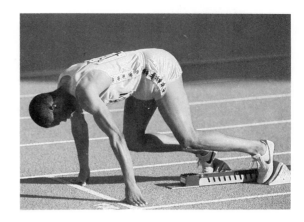

Calming down

People can feel 'threatened' by nice things too – the excitement before a party, the thrill of opening a longed-for present. It is adrenalin that tenses you up whenever your emotions are involved. But you cannot stay tensed up forever. Once the fear or challenge is over, another part of the 'fight or flight' system switches on to calm you down. Adrenalin stops pouring out, breathing and heart rate return to normal, and things like digestion start up again.

What is anxiety?

Anxiety is mild fear from inner challenges. 'Do I look all right? Will people like me?' and so on. Everyone has anxious moments about themselves now and then. A little anxiety is useful as it keys people up to do better. But anxiety can be harmful when it becomes a habit – a non-stop worrying and nagging inside the person's mind. People who stay anxious can become unhappy and tense. They risk losing their sense of well-being (p. 60).

Self help

Some people enjoy feeling slightly anxious and tense. They thrive on inner challenges. Other people do not. If you are a slightly anxious person and you don't enjoy it, try making a list of your problems. Then go down the list and see if worrying has made any of them better – *honestly*? Relax. Learn to talk your anxieties away. Talking really does help: keeping quiet does not. For further suggestions on how to cope with inner tensions, turn to page 74.

Questions

1 **What is the name of the 'fear' hormone?**
2 **List the ways in which adrenalin affects the whole body.**
3 **What is meant by the 'fight or flight' system?**
4 **Write about a time when you felt threatened and the 'fight or flight' system helped you.**
5 **'Fear is an important emotion'. Do you agree? What might happen if a person had no fear?**
6 **Explain what happens to your body once the danger is over.**
7 **In what ways can anxiety be (a) helpful and (b) harmful? Write a short essay, giving examples of each.**

Anger

What makes you angry? Is it when you cannot have your own way – perhaps not being allowed out, or not able to buy something you want? Or do you only get angry when you are unjustly accused – perhaps being told off for something you did not do? Try to remember when you were last angry. How did you feel?

Anger and adrenalin

Adrenalin is not just the 'fear' hormone. If floods through your body when you are angry too. But there are times when anger can be a dangerous emotion. Your intelligence knows you can make matters worse by 'blowing your top'. There are choices you can make. Study the three ways Jim dealt with anger when an unfair call was given against him on the football field.

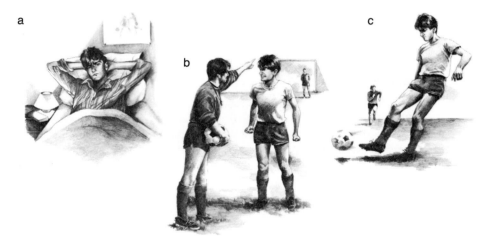

a Jim **suppressed** (held in) his anger. He raged and fumed inwardly. He went over and over what had happened – he wouldn't calm down. That night, he didn't sleep well. He woke late the next day. From then on, he blamed everything which went wrong on the unjust referee.

b Jim **expressed** (showed) his anger. He shouted and stormed. He yelled at the other players and he called the referee names. He was pleased when the others got angry and he enjoyed watching the referee go red in the face. He was sent off the field and banned from playing for the next two weeks.

c Jim **channelled** (let out safely) his anger. He said nothing, though he was furious inside. Once the game started again, he charged around the field and kicked the ball harder and straighter than he had ever managed before. By the end of the game, he had completely calmed down.

1 **Suppressed** (held in) anger may not be good for you if you let the fires of rage go on burning inside. You will become very tense.

2 **Expressed** (shown) anger may be good for you but bad for the people you pour your rage over. They may become very tense.

3 **Channelled** (let out safely) anger is usually the best choice. But anger is a powerful emotion, and this is not always easy. It takes a lot of practice, a lot of self-control and even more common sense!

4 Rational (reasoned) anger means you have a just cause and might make things better. Note that in the last example though Jim had a just cause he didn't argue with the referee. Can you work out the reasons why?

What is depression?

Mild depression is anger which is turned against yourself. 'Life is hard, unfair and cruel. I am useless. I cannot cope.' When things go wrong, everyone feels a bit useless from time to time – but they learn to cheer up. Depression is harmful when it becomes a habit – a non-stop brooding over past insults, injustices, and hurts. People who stay depressed can become unhappy and tense. They begin to believe that they, and life, are not worthwhile (p. 60).

Too much adrenalin?

Just as there are some fears you cannot fight or run away from (p. 69), so there are times when you cannot give way to anger. If people do not learn to cope with anger or fear, the extra energy which adrenalin has released is not used up. There is a risk this pent-up energy turns into a nasty frustrated sort of tension called **stress**. This means the body is constantly tensed for action, and the mind cannot relax. Too much stress going on for too long can cause physical (p. 95) as well as mental illness (p. 88).

Self help

1 Teach yourself to relax and unwind. This is easier said than done!

2 Remember you have choices about what to do with your anger. Count up to ten before you decide.

3 Vigorous exercise can channel angry feelings into safe places.

4 You can work them away too. Try scrubbing the floor, clearing out your room, or doing extra study.

5 Do your best not to brood. This keeps the painful feelings going on and on, and stops you cheering up.

6 If you sometimes feel tense for no particular reason, take up yoga or meditation to soothe your body and your mind.

7 Accept that anger and fear are natural parts of life, and learn how to cope with them in the best way to suit *you*.

Questions

1 **'Anger can be a dangerous emotion.' Do you agree, or not? Give reasons for your answer.**

2 **Copy into your book the choices you can make when you are angry.**

3 **What is stress? Name which of the suggestions in 'Self help' might best suit *you*.**

4 **Have a discussion on really wanting to lose your temper, but being able to hold it in check.**

Different kinds of behaviour

Imagine you are giving a party. The sausage rolls are on a plate under the grill. You pick up the plate. It is hot.

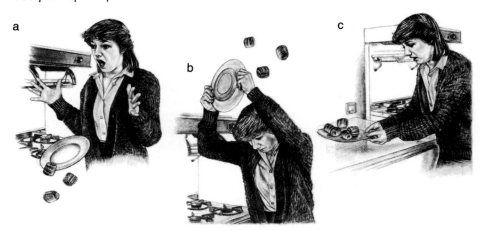

a   *Your mind is busy deciding what music to put on. Without thinking, you drop the hot plate. The sausage rolls are smashed to little bits.*

b   *You are cross because your favourite guest can't come. Burning your fingers is the last straw. You hurl the plate to the floor.*

c   *Your guests will be hungry. You haven't spent time and money for nothing. You hold on to the plate, but rush to put it safely down.*

What do you think *you* might have done in this situation?

Instinctive behaviour There are rare times when an action is purely instinctive. This is to protect you from harm.

Emotional behaviour There are times when your emotions are in control. You act impulsively (emotionally), whether it helps you or not.

Intelligent behaviour As you learn to reason things out, your actions become controlled by your intelligence. You act in the way which will help you most, no matter what your instincts or emotions tell you.

Behaviour

Behaviour is what you do – the way you act and react. Your emotions and intelligence show in the way you behave. If some people *always* acted intelligently and other people *always* acted emotionally, it would be easy to understand behaviour. But people chop and change from one kind of behaviour to the other. As you can see from the example above, it depends upon the situation.

Childish behaviour

Babies cry for food, warmth, comfort, and company. Toddlers throw temper tantrums when they can't get their own way. Four-year-old Zack is frightened of his play group. He whines and clings to his mother, begging her to stay. Children are ruled by their emotions. They cannot help behaving 'childishly'. They have only begun to think, to reason, to know, to understand. It takes a long time and a lot of practice to learn to act with intelligence. Most people spend most of their lives making choices between the two.

Mature behaviour

The older people get, the more they can reason out their behaviour. This is due to many things. Some of them are:

1 Mature people are more used to their emotions, and know which ones they can trust and which ones might let them down.
2 They have had lots of time to learn to reason out their behaviour.
3 They have made many mistakes, and hope to learn from them.
4 They have had lots of practice at coping with the negative emotions.

In spite of these things, adults are often ruled by their emotions. The point is, they *try* to keep the negative ones under some sort of intelligent control. For example: Mother Theresa (p. 67) didn't just sit down and weep with passionate pity for the poor. She used her intelligence to work passionately hard to improve their lives. You can see that behaviour can be both emotional *and* intelligent at the same time.

Keeping your emotions under some sort of intelligent control is a big part of what growing up and becoming an adult is about. This can start at any age – from seven to seventy!

'I couldn't help myself'

People say 'I couldn't help myself' all the time. And very often, it is true. There is nothing 'wrong' in being ruled by your emotions. It depends upon the situation you are in. Discuss the following tales thoroughly. Each person insisted that they couldn't help themselves. What do you think? Why do you think it is important that their ages are included?

1 Five-year-old Suzy is caught with a cream bun in her mouth.
2 Eleven-year-old Johnny nearly drowns when he jumps into the river and rescues his friend.
3 Fourteen-year-old Tom has to appear in a Juvenile Court for taking and driving away a car.
4 Nineteen-year-old Mary loses her well-paid job when she tells off the manager for making racist remarks.
5 Twenty-year-old Gary is pulled out from the middle of a football riot with an opened flick-knife in his hand.

Questions

1 **Copy out the definition of 'emotional behaviour'.**
2 **Do you think people who act with intelligence are 'cold fish'? Give reasons for your answer.**
3 **Make up two short stories, one with a happy ending and the other with a sad ending, in which both emotional and intelligent behaviour are used at the same time.**
4 **Turn to page 118 and study the two lists. Discuss them.**

Choices and conflicts

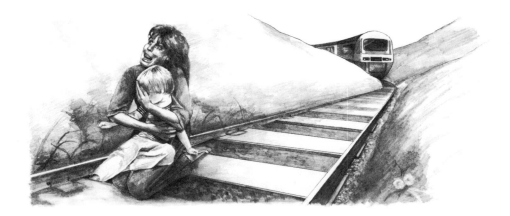

'A little boy caught his foot under the railway line. A train was coming near. His mother tried desperately to save him, but he was trapped. In tears, she ran to the side to save her own life. But when she saw the terror on her child's face, she knew she couldn't leave him to die alone. She ran back. Shielding him with her body from the oncoming train, she held him in her arms – and waited.'

Think about this true story. The mother had two other small children at home. What happened to her instinct for self-preservation? Her other children needed her. What happened to her intelligence? You may think she was foolish, or the story may touch you deeply – perhaps a little of both. But you will certainly see the power of human emotions, and the choices people are free to make.

Choices

Mark wakes up in a bad mood. Will he choose to make the best of things – or the worst? Will he rise early, wash and tidy himself and greet the family cheerfully? Or rise late, neglect his appearance and give everyone grumpy looks?

Choices are fascinating. People make them all the time. Mark's choices were simple. But many choices are very difficult. Some seem almost impossible to make.

Judy and her friends are caught truanting from school. Judy is asked for an explanation. Should she make up a lie to get herself and her friends out of trouble? Or tell the truth, which will land all of them in a mess?

Conflicts

Judy is torn between her instincts, her emotions and her intelligence. Her instincts tell her to get out of trouble. Her emotions tell her to protect her friends. Her intelligence tells her that she doesn't like lying and she thinks people who tell lies are not worthwhile. This kind of **inner conflict** keeps happening to people. It is like a battle being fought in the mind. Each person has to fight for her or himself in choosing between very conflicting choices. Which choice do you think might suit Judy best?

The truth?

Judy tells the truth. Her friends are cross and won't speak to her. They all have to spend a week in detention. 'You told the truth,' her father comforts her. 'It is always quicker in the long run.' As Judy waits miserably for the week to end so that she can make it up with her friends, she wonders: 'Is telling the truth really quicker?' What do you think?

The lie?

Judy makes up a lie. Her friends are admiring: 'Ooh, we wouldn't have dared!' Judy is angry; she only only did it for them. To make matters worse, though the teacher says nothing, Judy believes he knows she was lying. She can't bear to look at him. She hates being thought a liar. To protect herself from these painful feelings, Judy pretends she has stopped liking the teacher. She starts handing in poor work. Each week as his lesson comes round, Judy feels more miserable, more angry and more tense. From one inner conflict, she has now many more.

Conscience

Your conscience also controls your behaviour. It is your moral guide. It helps you to choose the things you think are right, and not to choose the things you think are wrong. People do not like to think of themselves as liars or thieves. Your conscience isn't just your moral guide. It helps to keep you liking yourself and feeling you are worthwhile – mentally healthy. What do you think Judy can do to stop her inner conflicts and mental pain? Have a discussion on this.

Summary

1 The emotions are a powerful drive in human behaviour.
2 They can overcome the instincts and the intelligence.
3 They can be a force for great good or great evil; they will make you happy or miserable – depending on how you use them.
4 This also holds true for the intelligence and the choices you make.
5 Choices and conflicts are part of being human. Mental health and happiness depends upon some kind of balance between the two.

Self help

People make choices they know are wrong for lots of different reasons. During the teens these reasons may include wanting to shock, or to please. Have you been in a situation rather like Judy's? Try to work out the reason why, and whether you made the best choice in the long run for *you*.

Questions

1 **Read the story of the boy and mother again. Do you think the mother's behaviour heroic, or foolish? Give reasons for your answer.**
2 **In what ways does the story show that the emotions can overcome the instincts and the intelligence?**
3 **The results of Judy's choices are imaginary. Make up two other scenes which might have happened as the result of Judy's choices.**
4 **'People are free to make choices about their behaviour.' Discuss this statement. Can you think of examples where this may not be true?**

About attitudes

Are you an optimist, or a pessimist? Look at the glass of orange juice.

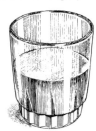

'The glass is half empty,' says the pessimist.
'The glass is half full,' says the optimist.

The pessimist has a negative attitude to life, always looking for the worst side. The optimist has a positive attitude, always looking for the best. As love can be called a 'health cocktail', so too can optimism. Optimism is about hope, and everyone needs the power of hope.

Why hope?

Life is not always happy. Things can and do go wrong. This means people cannot expect to feel 'good' all the time. But during the 'bad times' people with positive attitudes have the strength to soldier on, to hope for better days. The pessimist may feel swamped by misery, and suffer terrible despair.

What are attitudes?

Attitudes are your ways of feeling and thinking about life. They come from your emotions and your intelligence, and from what you have learned in the past. They form an important part of your character as they 'colour' (affect) almost everything you say or do. People who lead happy, contented lives always have a positive attitude towards themselves and life.

Your real attitudes

Most people are neither wild optimists, nor wild pessimists. They are somewhere in between. In fact, many people who sound negative are quite the opposite – see p. 60. They get a gloomy enjoyment from being mournful. They say, 'Of course I've failed the exam', so that if they pass, they can be even more delighted; if they fail, they do not have to be too unhappy. Their attitude is the same as the optimist – *positive*. Are you a secret optimist?

Attitudes as habits

From quite an early age, people develop habits of thinking positively or negatively about themselves. Over the years, these habits of thinking may harden and people's attitudes can become set. Do you know any person who always expects the worst, or the best? Which kind of person would you rather be?

During the teens, your whole way of thinking may be shaken up as you learn to look at life from other points of view. If you do not like your attitudes, now is the time to change – before you get set in your ways!

Negative attitudes

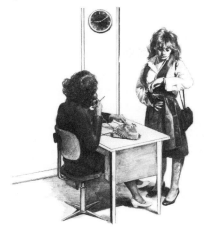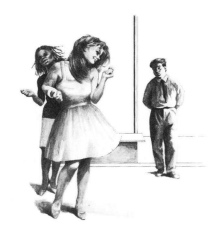

'I won't get that job. I just know I won't.' Janice doesn't bother with her appearance and arrives late for the interview.

'If I ask her to dance, I just know she'll turn me down.' Steven stays at the back of the hall and has a miserable evening.

Both Janice and Steven deliberately set out to fail. Have a discussion on why you think they do this. Fears of failing can be very painful, but neither person can win anything if they don't try. Negative attitudes which stop people doing their best are not likely to lead to a happy and contented life.

Finding out:
What you think are positive and negative attitudes.

Put the following words into two lists under the headings *Positive* and *Negative*. When you have finished, compare your lists with a friend. Do you both agree, or not?

kind	admiring	depressed	confident
timid	pessimistic	brave	intolerant
tolerant	mean	unfair	dishonest
fair	truthful	spiteful	generous
envious	over-anxious	optimistic	hopeful

Questions

1 **What is meant by 'a negative attitude to life'?**
2 **Write down three words which might describe an optimist.**
3 **In your own words, explain the importance of hope.**
4 **'Attitudes are states of mind.' Using the text, explain what this means.**
5 **What advice would you give a friend who wants to break the habit of having spiteful and mean thoughts?**
6 **Role-play what you would do in either Janice's or Steven's place.**

About the unconscious mind

There are two levels at which the mind works: the conscious level, where you know what is going on, and the unconscious level, where you do not. The unconscious mind used to be called the *sub*conscious because it works *below* or *underneath* the level of the conscious mind.

Past memories are stored in the unconscious, many of which your thinking mind has forgotten. There are happy memories – the candles on your second birthday cake, and unhappy memories – the jealousy you felt when a baby brother or sister was born. A few memories may be so dreadful (threatening) that your conscious mind blacked them out, refusing to admit they ever happened. They are locked away in your unconscious, but, every now and again, bits of the dreadfulness filter back. For a short while, you feel tense, angry, anxious, or miserable without knowing why. This usually happens when the same kind of threatening situation crops up again.

'Stop, thief!'

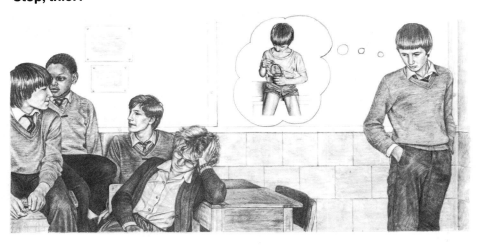

Money has been stolen from the cloakrooms. Everyone is asked to stay behind. The others wait; bored, irritated, or idly chatting. Adam isn't guilty, but he is seized with terrible feelings of panic and outrage. Do they think he is a thief? How *dare* they!

Adam does not remember stealing from his mother's purse when he was seven. He felt so guilty that the sweets he bought made him sick, and he completely blacked the memory from his conscious mind. Adam is now very intolerant of people who steal. He thinks they are wicked and should have their hands chopped off.

When our conscious mind cannot accept 'bad' things about ourselves, our unconscious puts these 'bad' feelings onto other people. This is called **projection**. A study of the people you most dislike may well give you insight into your own buried memories – those things which make you angry or anxious without knowing why.

The personality

People say things like: 'She's got her Dad's fiery temper but she's not a bit like him otherwise.' Not enough is yet known about whether we inherit bits of our personality from our parents (p. 144). But it seems likely that we do, and that they are stored in the unconscious. The unconscious stores other information about us too – such things as our attitudes (p. 76) and our moral guides (p. 75). Over the years, all this stored information comes together to help form the **personality** – the kind of people we become.

The unconscious works hard to keep us 'true' to our personality. It seeks *peace* and *harmony* with the conscious thinking mind. Often it loses. We are likely to behave 'against' our personalities when we feel threatened by unpleasant situations. For people like Judy (p. 74) and Adam, this causes a lot of inner conflicts and a lot of mental pain.

Mental aches and pains

Remember that the psyche is the whole mind, conscious and unconscious. The psyche can be 'bruised' in much the same way as the body can. We all get knocks to our pride. We fear being unloved, or not being 'good' enough. Suppressed angers and anxieties can suddenly flare up (p. 70). This is part of being human, and just as bruises on the body take a while to fade, so bruises on the psyche also take a while to heal. But there are certain times when we can speed up this healing. These are when the aches and pains are caused by inner conflicts such as Judy's and Adam's.

Know thyself!

If Adam had owned up when he was seven, his conscious mind would have accepted that he was *once* a thief but that didn't make him *always* a thief. Owning up helps people to forgive themselves, and to forget. Adam may still dislike thieves – who doesn't? – but he wouldn't feel so panicky and intolerant towards them. The psyche is self-healing if we can accept the 'bad' as well as the 'good' sides of our personalities. The more you learn about yourself and act in the best way for *you*, the less likely you are to get into the sort of muddles Judy *unconsciously* built for herself.

Questions

1 **Name the two levels at which the mind works.**
2 **The unconscious used to be called the subconscious. Explain why.**
3 **Happy memories can also filter back from the unconscious. If this has happened to you, try to work out the connection between the past and now.**
4 **'When we try to be what we are not, or we fail to be what we are – the psyche is in trouble.' Write a short essay about this statement.**
5 **'No deed is so wicked it cannot be forgiven.' Do you agree, or disagree? Have a discussion about this.**
6 **Without giving away personal secrets, write about a time when you did something wrong which made you feel quite ill afterwards. Perhaps choose an incident which happened when you were young.**

Sleep and dreams

You spend almost a third of your life with your conscious mind switched off. During sleep, your heart beat slows down, your muscles lose tone, and even your eyes relax, turning upward and outward under closed lids. The body's work, such as the production of saliva, tears, and urine, slows down too.

Some people need far more sleep than others. During the teens, you may need stretches of extra long sleep. Your physical and mental development can be tiring. The average eight hours may not be enough!

Two kinds of sleep

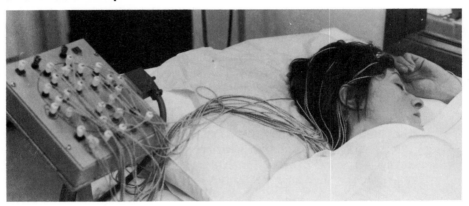

There are two kinds of sleep. In one, the growth hormone is released, new cells are built, and worn-out cells are removed. The other, called Rapid Eye Movement or REM, is the time when you dream. Some people insist they do not dream, but if a sleeper is woken during REM, the dream is clearly remembered. You need both kinds of sleep. They happen in turn right through the night.

Insomnia comes from the Latin (*somnus*, to sleep). It means being unable to sleep. Teenagers rarely suffer from this. Adults often do. The biggest cause of insomnia is anxiety, which in turn creates more anxiety over not sleeping. Sleeping drugs help, for a while. They do not, however, cure the anxiety which first triggered off the insomnia.

Dreams

Have you gone to bed with a problem and woken up knowing the answer? Each day, a lot of information pours into your mind. Some scientists think that during the night, your dreams sort it out. When the unconscious comes across the problem, it tries to work it out. But the unconscious doesn't use reason or logic, as the conscious mind does. It relies on past memories, imagination, and intuition; it 'thinks' in stories, parables, and symbols.

This is why dreams often don't seem to make sense. Your conscious mind thinks them nonsense – 'It's only a silly dream.' But the unconscious has been busy trying one solution after another, which is why the dream is always changing. When the unconscious does find the answer, 'sleep on it' turns out to be very good advice.

Nightmares

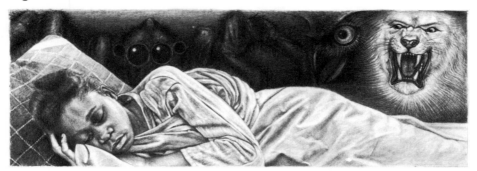

But problems do not always have easy answers. The dream can turn dark and terrifying. Horrid though nightmares are, they are still trying to help. They may give you shrewd insight into behaviour your conscious mind refuses to accept. A dream of dying might mean the death of your sense of feeling worthwhile. You have done something nasty and you hate yourself for it. You are being shown the conflict in your unconscious from one of your actions.

The recurring nightmare, a dream which comes back over and over again, is often due to fears left over from childhood. The unconscious keeps digging them up – usually at times of stress – to have another go at sorting them out. Even though this can be terribly upsetting, you can see how hard your unconscious works at trying to give you peace of mind. Recurring dreams usually stop in the late teens, as you grow more confident and assured.

Wish-fulfilment dreams

These are about the things you hope will happen in the future. Wish-fulfilment dreams are usually very nice: winning prizes, scoring goals, becoming famous and admired. But one or two can be horrid – a member of your family or a close friend is dying, or in great danger. This doesn't mean you *really* want that person to be harmed. The dream is helping you get rid of small revenges in a huge, magnified, very distorted way. Most people don't really want to be a member of the Royal Family. They just want to be admired and loved in the same way.

Self help

It takes most adults about twenty minutes to fall asleep. It will probably take you less. Go to bed before you become over-tired, and settle down with a cheerful book. Over-heated rooms and meals last thing at night can trigger off disturbing dreams. Think positively, not negatively, before you fall asleep.

Questions

1 **Write down three things which happen during sleep.**
2 **Name the two kinds of sleep, and explain what they are.**
3 **What is insomnia? Who suffers from it, and why?**
4 **In your own words, explain in what ways a nightmare can be trying to help.**
5 **Without giving away personal secrets, write about (a) a wish-fulfilment dream you have or (b) one you would like to have.**

About adolescent mental health (1)

There is no such person as a typical adolescent. But because the teens are the in-between stage, there are certain doubts and muddled feelings which may happen at times. Do you recognize any of the following?

1   Feeling wildly happy one moment, then miserable the next.
2   Worrying over looks, over being popular, over health.
3   Giving very strong opinions but not being able to explain them.
4   Having outbursts of temper followed by painful feelings of remorse.
5   Promising yourself to do better and despairing when you fail.
6   Being sure of yourself but feeling awkward and shy.
7   Making close loving friendships which suddenly go wrong.
8   Wanting to be like others (your peer group), but different as well.
9   Having very sensitive feelings but sometimes ignoring other people's.
10 Insisting on a private life without help or hindrance from adults.
11 Going right off authority; perhaps parents, teachers, or the law.
12 Wanting to improve the world but not knowing where or how to begin.
13 Having explosions of energy between long bouts of inertia.
14 At times, feeling utterly and totally and intensely bored.

This is the uncomfortable side of the teens. You feel full of restless energy. You want to get on with your life. But uncertainties and confusions keep cropping up – excited longings and fierce angers and horrid self-doubt. Adolescence is to do with the growth of your intelligence *and* your emotions. It isn't easy. You may be called 'touchy' or 'moody'. It is likely you are. No-one enjoys feeling uncertain of themselves. But teenage moods don't last long. They pass as quickly as they come.

Beware!

'Who needs friends?' thinks the lonely person. 'The others cheated,' thinks the loser. 'They're all against me,' thinks the person who is battling with authority. These are **defence mechanisms**: excuses made up by the unconscious to stop painful feelings. Everyone uses them now and then. They are comforting for a little while but because they are not true, the painful feelings go on. In time, the person admits they are excuses and learns to make friends, stop battling, or whatever. During intense emotional upset, beware of defence mechanisms. There is a risk you start believing them. You stop trying to sort things out.

Being positive

Sophie was training to be a ballet dancer. But at 15, she grew three more inches and was told she was too tall. For a while Sophie was in despair. She refused to work. She gave up her piano practice which she loved. Then, quite suddenly, she could hardly be dragged away from the piano. 'If I can't be a ballet dancer,' she muttered, 'I'll make sure I'm good at something.'

This defence mechanism is called **compensation**. We make up or compensate for losing one thing by replacing it with another. Compensation is a useful defence mechanism when it gets us out of the misery of failure and directs us towards a chance to succeed. Not all compensations are as dramatic as Sophie's.

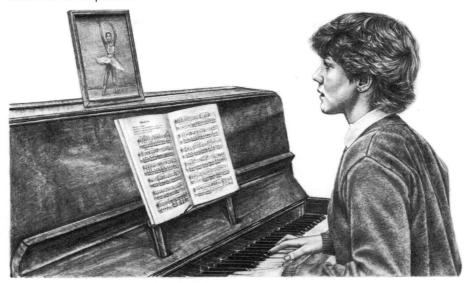

Look at the list again. It may seem very negative. But these doubts and confusions are part of the life force driving you forward. Without examining yourself and your world, you might never grow up. Try not to think, 'I can't wait to grow up' because now is the time to *grow through* your insecure feelings and to learn you can cope.

Self help

Calm down before you talk about your feelings. Talking things out really does help. Choose an adult whose opinions you respect, who can help you sort things out. When you feel 'touchy' or 'moody', retreat to your room and play music or whatever calms you down. Try not to battle with others – it is likely to make things worse, not better. You need calming times to learn you *can* control these feelings. Adolescence is as exciting as it is difficult. Remember the unsteady patches don't last for long.

Questions

1 **In what ways do you think you are (a) a typical adolescent and (b) an untypical one? Look again at the list, and note which points apply to you.**
2 **'People who are active in sport, music, drama, or other interests do not suffer boredom or bouts of inertia.' Write down reasons why this statement might be true.**
3 **In your own words, explain what is meant by a 'defence mechanism'. Make up or write down one of your own.**
4 **In what ways do defence mechanisms help people?**
5 **Explain how believing in a defence mechanism might actually harm you.**
6 **What advice would you give a person who says, 'I can't wait to grow up'? Give as many helpful points as you can.**

About adolescent mental health (2)

Becoming mature means being able to accept the person you really are, and to understand the world as it really is. Below are some skills to help you learn how to cope.

Self-fulfilment

Make a list of your **needs** – the big, important things in life. (New clothes or a television set are 'wants' rather than needs. You can get along without them if you have to.)

The fulfilment of your needs is what you should work towards. This may sound selfish, but your goals are not narrow. To be happy you need to be committed (totally involved); not only to yourself but to others and the rest of your world.

The future

Work for your future. Whatever the state of employment, you need to have some skills. Study hard for them. Whether you are bright or not, concentrate on all the things which make up your intelligence. Will-power, self-control, judgement, sensitivity, and stamina are very important in all aspects of your life. They give you confidence and improve the way you feel about yourself.

The present

If you have developed a habit of feeling 'bad', *learn to like yourself*. Not in a silly boasting way, but deep down where you really are nice. Forget those feelings of being worthless or useless. You are not, and the future will prove you right. Throw away self-pity, it will only hold you back.

Keep remembering your good points – the kind things you have done and intend to do in the future; the parts of your character which make you special and worthwhile. Concentrate very hard on this and you will notice results. The more you like yourself, the more others will like you too.

'Alter or adjust'

Everyone has problems; it helps to remember that. Draw up a list of your problems: study? work? family arguments? self-image? lack of friends? Examine the list carefully, then start to 'alter or adjust'.

1 If you dislike the situation, do your best to alter it (change it).
2 If you can't alter the situation, do you best to adjust (change yourself).

These are the two golden rules on how to solve problems.

Think about these examples:

There is a risk of lead in your hot-water pipe:
'That's not my fault', says A, filling the kettle from the hot tap.
'I'll join the anti-lead lobby,' says B, and uses the cold tap.

Quarrelling makes you angry and tense:
'They started it,' says A, going red in the face and scowling.
'Let's agree to differ,' says B, and begins to calm down.

Do you think A or B is more likely to be at peace with themselves, other people and their world?

During the teens, it isn't always possible to alter a situation. Nor may you be the best judge of whether the situation really *should* be altered. But this is put as the first golden rule so that you can remember it later on. Also, this first rule applies to inner conflicts: 'When you try to be what you are not, or you fail to be what you are – the psyche is in trouble.' Sort out your inner problems by learning more about yourself, *then* adapt to those you can do nothing about. For example: if you know you are lazy, accept this as part of yourself, then adapt to it by setting yourself certain tasks and *checking that you do them*. (Don't make these tasks too difficult or you might fail!)

Remember, you are striving towards harmony and peace of mind – an inner wholeness; and you are striving towards a satisfactory relationship between yourself and others, and the world you live in. Many psychiatrists and philosophers believe these strivings are innate (inborn) in all humans.

Summary

1 Mental health comes from a sense of well-being, from having worthwhile goals and working hard to achieve them.
2 Material comforts are 'wants' rather than 'needs' and do not on their own make people happy or add to the meaning of life.
3 Learn to 'alter or adjust'. Don't give up at your failures. Take pleasure when you win.
4 Train yourself to think positively, not negatively – you can do it if you try!
5 Don't take yourself too solemnly. Mental health is about being happy.

Questions

1 **Name two things a mature person is able to do.**
2 **Self-fulfilment sounds dreadfully selfish. In as much detail as you can, explain why it is not.**
3 **'Intelligence is far more than passing exams.' Give examples of at least three other things you need for a happy life.**
4 **In what ways can people change habits of feeling 'bad'? Why do you think it is important they do change?**
5 **In your own words, explain what is meant by 'alter or adjust'. Think up and write down an example of your own.**
6 **Describe what you think is meant by a 'well-adjusted' person.**
7 **Copy out the summary. Learn the points with which you agree.**

Early emotional development

The baby

A baby has times of wild excitements and joys. He also has times when he feels very distressed. He chuckles and gurgles during his happy times. He cries when he needs food, company, or warmth. A baby cannot bear to feel 'bad'. He is too little to cope with distress. For the healthy development of his emotions, he needs to feel 'good' for most of the time.

Helping the baby's emotional development

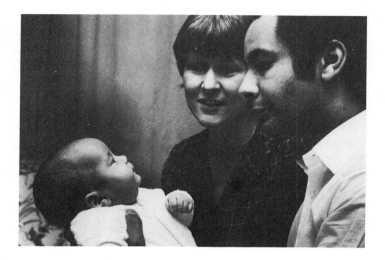

Most parents do their best to take away a baby's bad feelings. They pick him up when he cries, and try to put things right. The baby quickly learns he is important to these people because when he feels bad they come and make him feel good again. He loves and trusts his parents. He develops a sense of well-being. He feels worthwhile, good about himself and other people, and able to face the challenges of life.

Harming the baby's emotional development

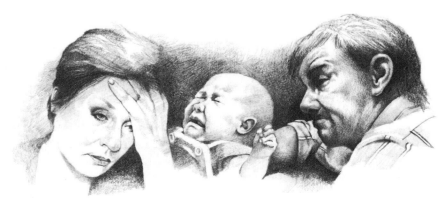

A few parents do not understand the importance of a baby's feelings. They expect the baby to wait for what he needs, as if he were grown-up. The baby quickly learns he is not very important to these people because when he feels bad they do not help him feel good again. He loves but distrusts his parents. He develops anxious feelings that all is far from well. He feels worthless, bad about himself and other people, and not able to face the challenges of life.

Why a baby's feelings are so important

You can see that things can go wrong very early in life. And nowadays, it is believed that those first emotional experiences remain with the person for life: that by the time a child is three years old, the memory patterns for emotional attitudes and behaviour are laid down and developed.

You may understand this better if you think about the memory patterns for walking. The adult does not have to remember how to walk. The memory patterns were laid down and developed during the toddler stage – walking is now a habit. Much the same thing happens with the emotions – feeling 'good' or 'bad' becomes a habit. This is *not* the same as being a secret optimist (p. 76). Babies are no different from the rest of us. They have an inborn drive to be happy – to feel good.

1   It is unlikely any baby feels totally unloved the whole time. But raising a child is not easy. Nearly all parents make a few mistakes.
2   A few mistakes don't matter. Children laugh them off when they grow up as their parents did before them.
3   However, too many mistakes over emotional development can turn a happy baby into an anxious or depressed adult (p. 71).
4   All babies need love, security, praise, and encouragement to help them develop a sense of well-being.

Community help

Parents, especially mothers on their own, can get tired and need a break from their children. Why not help? If you don't know any parents, go to a clinic or Child Health Centre and offer your services – baby minding, pram pushing at the weekends, taking toddlers to the Zoo, or whatever you feel you could do to help.

Questions

1   **How does a baby show he is (a) happy, (b) unhappy?**
2   **Write down three things which happen to a baby whose parents are helpful.**
3   **In your own words, explain why a baby's early emotional experiences are so important.**
4   **Write about a few of the things which can go wrong in early emotional development.**
5   **'All future parents should be taught Child Development.' Do you agree? Give reasons for your answer.**

About mental illness (1)

Until quite recently, people found it difficult to believe in mental illness. People were either 'possessed by devils' or something was physically wrong with their 'nerves'. We still use the terms 'nervous breakdown' and 'nervous disorder' but in nearly all mental illness there is nothing wrong with people's nerves.

People were frightened of mental illness. It was seen as a mark of weakness and a terrible family disgrace. Mentally ill people were often treated cruelly, hidden away or locked in lunatic asylums. Lunatic comes from the Latin (*luna*, the moon) as people were supposed to be affected by the moon. Even today, unkind words like 'loonies' and 'weirdos' are used; books and films are still produced which carry on this notion. Of course the mind can get ill, just as the body can.

What is mental illness?

It is even more difficult to define mental illness than to define mental health. Perhaps it is best to think of mental illness as '*ordinary* feelings which become so *intense*, so *exaggerated*, and so *out-of-proportion* that the person *cannot* cope with them'. It is no use saying to a mentally ill person, 'pull yourself together' or 'snap out of it'. He or she has lost all sense of well-being, and cannot. Proper medical help is needed.

Can mental illness be cured?

Yes. Just as the body can be treated and cured, so can the mind. And in the same way, early treatment is far better than late. This is especially true of mental illness, as the person often suffers great agony of mind. The longer the pain goes on, the worse the illness is likely to become.

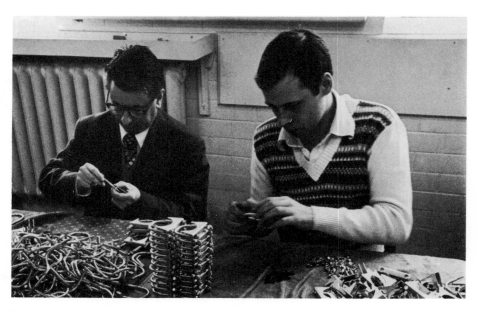

The people working here are recovering from mental illnesses.

Self-image and stress

Your self-image is how you 'see' (think and feel about) yourself. You read about stress on page 71. Everyone has some stress in their lives. We all suffer from things going wrong, and from anger, jealousy, pride, greed, fear of failing, or not liking ourselves now and then. People with a sense of well-being use stress as a challenge to help them do better, and to alter or adjust. It is the adult with too many inner conflicts, and perhaps a low self-image, who is likely to be overwhelmed and break down under stress.

The facts

1 Mental illness is increasing. It is a major health problem today.
2 One in ten adults will spend some time in a psychiatric hospital.
3 One third of hospital beds are for the mentally ill, while thousands more are treated at home by their family doctors.
4 Many emotional disorders can be traced back to 'bad' early childhood experiences. Parents need help to avoid these mistakes.
5 Schools should do more to educate adolescents in understanding their emotional needs and learning how to cope with their problems.
6 It is now believed most mental illness could have been avoided, and nearly all can be treated – even when the illness has become serious.

Community help

A residential home is being planned for people recovering from mental illness. The local residents are trying to stop this. They say the value of their properties will go down. They insist the home should be built elsewhere. Have a discussion on this.

Finding out:
The work of MIND.

This is the National Association for Mental Health. Write to them, enclosing a stamped addressed envelope, for details of their work. Choose one topic and do a full project on it.

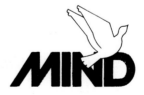

Questions

1 **'It is still more acceptable to be physically ill than mentally ill.' Do you agree? Give reasons for your answer.**
2 **Copy out the definition of mental illness.**
3 **Write about three of the problems which might cause people stress.**
4 **Explain why stress on its own does not always cause mental illness.**
5 **'Most mental illness could have been avoided.' Explain why all parents-to-be, and everyone working with small children, should be taught how to develop a sense of well-being and a positive self-image in the child.**

About mental illness (2)

The psychoses

A psychosis is any mental illness where the person loses touch with reality. These are very serious illnesses. The most common is **schizophrenia**. This means 'split mind' and there are many different kinds. But in all kinds the person, finding life unbearably painful, withdraws into a fantasy world. Other people cannot make contact. The person usually does not know he is ill. His behaviour may be violent or 'frozen'. He needs urgent medical help.

The neuroses

These are far less serious because the person does not lose touch with reality. But this can make life even more painful. Too much mental pain will make the 'toughest' person break. **Tranquillizers** and **anti-depressants** are the drugs used to calm or block off the painful emotions. The person is helped to find the cause of this unhappiness.

Anxiety states When feelings of anxiety turn into intense panic. These people feel so threatened by inner fears they are unable to calm down. Nor can these fears be explained away by reason; they cannot see they are out of proportion. They are overwhelmed by intense anxiety.

Depression When feelings of despair take over completely. This may happen after a betrayal, a failure, a let-down. As the person believes there is no help left in life, there seems no point in trying. They become dulled and inactive, unable to look after themselves or others.

Phobias Extreme fear of open or closed spaces, or crowds, or noise, or heights, and so on. These people feel they must constantly be on guard against these threats. They cannot get on with their lives as they are unable to relax.

Obsessions These are frantic needs to check and re-check, or to repeat certain actions over and over again. These people are driven by inner compulsions they cannot control. They are unable to move forward with life as they are caught in a circle of repeated thought or action.

It is not unusual during the teens for people to wonder if their intense feelings are a sign of neurotic illness. Anger, anxiety, guilt, depression: these are perfectly normal feelings everyone has when things go wrong. But in a neurotic illness these emotions become so *extreme* and so *unending* they take over the person's whole life. They do not come and go like ordinary unhappy feelings. They are there, the whole time, like a fever of the mind. And as a feverish person cannot laugh or chatter or enjoy watching television, so a person suffering a neurotic illness cannot do these things either.

Treatment of the neuroses

1 **Psychoanalysis** People are helped to discover *for themselves* the conflicts and fears which are buried in their unconscious. They then analyse them, and learn how to cope with them. This can be a long and difficult method.

2 **Psychotherapy** People are helped to face *their own* fears, often by working in groups. Each person's problems are discussed openly and the group gives advice. Psychotherapy often works by giving people a better insight into their own problems by understanding the problems of others.

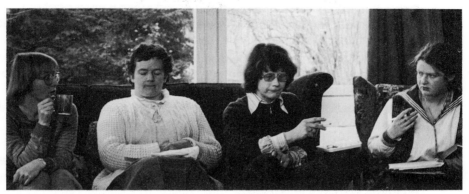

A group therapy session

Psychosomatic illness

Soma means body. A psychosomatic illness is a real physical illness partly caused or made worse by mental stress. Certain kinds of heart disease, stomach troubles, skin rashes, and migraines (headaches) are among these illnesses.

Community help

People are different. Some are naturally far more sensitive than others. What may seem like a little mild teasing on your part could be causing intense mental pain. Adolescents can be surprisingly cruel in their teasing – without realizing its effect. Have you teased anyone recently? What was it about?

Remember, people need to be able to:
like themselves and feel worthwhile;
feel good about others;
face up to the bad as well as the good sides of life.

Questions

1 **What is the most usual psychosis? What does the name mean?**
2 **Why may a neurotic illness be even more painful than a psychotic one?**
3 **Name the two groups of drugs used to treat a neurosis.**
4 **Look up the meanings of 'agoraphobia' and 'claustrophobia'. Write two sentences which show you understand the meaning of each word.**
5 **'If you walk in the squares, you won't be eaten by bears.' Small children play the game of not being able to step on lines. Can you remember any harmless obsessive game you played?**
6 **In what ways would you know your intense feelings were not a sign of mental illness?**

Further work on Chapter 2

1 Dab a thin film of paint on your fingers and make a copy of your fingerprints. Compare them with a friend's. How does the 'difference' show that comparisons between people don't mean much?

2 Adults motivate children to do difficult tasks. At what stage in life do you think people can motivate themselves? Give one example you have noticed to illustrate your answer.

3 At 16, Jan is doing very well at school but she is romantically in love and wants to get married. She asks your advice. What would you say?

4 Do a full project on the work of Mother Theresa of Calcutta.

5 'A few teenagers are show-offs and very boastful. They are only interested in *getting* pleasure (self-love).' Have a discussion on whether you agree or disagree with this statement.

6 Have you ever suppressed (a) giggles, (b) a rude remark, and (c) tears of temper? In each case say why it was necessary, and what helped you to do this. (For example: you may suppress giggles in order not to hurt someone else's feelings.)

7 A friend is a bit depressed over failing an exam. What would you say to cheer them up and make them feel worthwhile again?

8 Without giving away personal secrets, describe a time when you acted impulsively (emotionally) (a) with painful results and (b) with very satisfactory results.

9 'Don't be childish!' people sometimes say. In terms of emotional and intelligent behaviour, what do they mean?

10 Judy's lie made her feel unhappy and tense (p. 74). Imagine all the people in your neighbourhood suddenly lost their conscience. Would life be more, or less, peaceful? Give examples to illustrate your answer.

11 'Laugh, and the world laughs with you. Weep, and you weep alone.' In what ways do you think this might apply to (a) the optimist and (b) the pessimist?

12 In groups, make a list of lots of possible defence mechanisms. Then, on your own, try to think which ones might apply to you.

13 Being able to laugh at mistakes helps people to avoid getting anxious or depressed. Do you agree, or disagree? Think up some examples to include in your reply.

14 Find the address of your local Samaritans in the telephone directory. Write or pay them a visit. Do a full project on their work.

15 Write a full essay describing some of the ways in which learning to alter or adjust can help people keep their sense of well-being.

Chapter 3

About the top killers

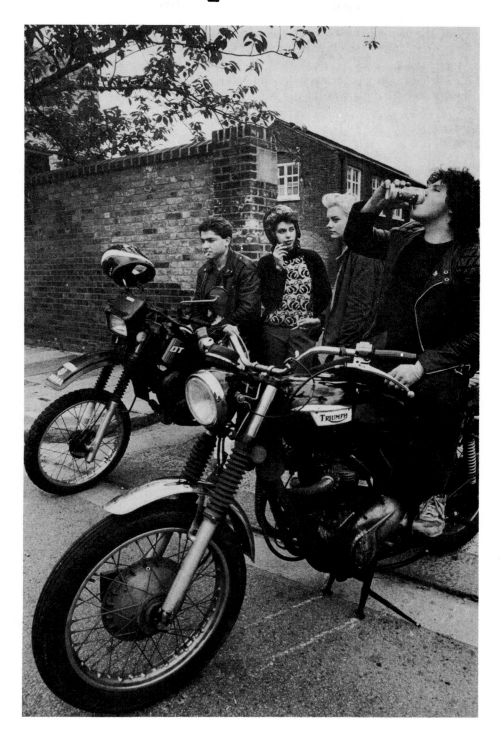

About heart disease

Today's top killers

A hundred years ago, the top killers were infectious diseases. Since then, great improvements in diet, hygiene, and health care have almost wiped them out. Today's top killers are heart disease, bronchitis, cancer, and accidents. Deaths from or related to alcohol, smoking, and drug abuse are high on the list. Like the infectious diseases, many of these deaths can be avoided. Preventive action can be taken now.

Your heart

Your heart is a magnificent pump. It started beating about eight months before you were born and will go on, without rest, until the end of your life. It is made of **cardiac** muscle, special muscle which is not under the control of your will. Its work is to pump blood through tubes called **arteries** and **veins** to all parts of your body.

Your heart and exercise

Your heart beats about 100,000 times a day. During the average life, it beats a least 2,500 million times. Heart is nearly all muscle – and muscle gets stronger and fitter with exercise, weaker and feebler without. During the teens, heart weight nearly doubles and it is now you build up strong sturdy cardiac muscle to last you for life.

Your heart and diet

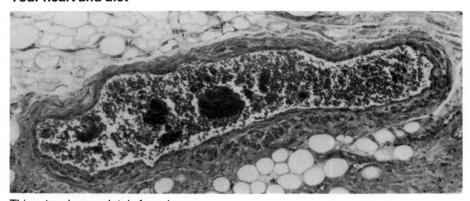

This artery is completely furred up.

Cholesterol comes from food rich in animal fats (p. 43). If there is too much cholesterol in the blood, it can stick to the inside of the arteries in tiny patches. This causes the arteries to narrow and 'fur up'. If the tiny patches flake off – like rust in a pipe – they can form a clot where the artery wall is rough or damaged. Narrow arteries and blood clots cause heart attacks and strokes (p. 38).

Smoking also narrows the arteries by causing the fats to stick to the sides.

Eating too many sugary foods can make you overweight. This extra burden can put unnecessary strain on the heart.

Blood pressure

This is the force at which the heart pumps blood into the arteries. If the arteries are damaged, the blood pressure can rise. Older people may have high blood pressure; it can be safely lowered by drugs. You can record your heart beat at pressure points called **pulses**. The usual place to take the pulse is at the wrist.

Normal pulse rates are: Adults: 80–60 beats per minute. Newborn: 140–120. I to 3 year olds: 120–90. 7 to 14 year olds: 90–80. 14 to 20 year olds: 70+.

During exercise and strong emotion, the rate of your heart beat rises. It quickly returns to normal when your mind or body relaxes. But if a person stays tensed up – angry or fearful – then the body stays tense too. The heart is under extra strain, ready for flight or fight (p. 68). This is why too much worry and stress is bad for the heart. Heart disease accounts for a third of all deaths.

Self help

1 Grill food, don't fry it. Cut right down on cholesterol foods (p. 43).
2 Do not begin smoking. If you already have, try to stop (p. 99).
3 Keep active. You need vigorous exercise throughout life (p. 32).
4 Try relaxation classes if you need to cut down worry and stress (p. 71).
5 Keep your weight fairly steady. Overweight strains the heart (p. 47).
6 These self-help guidelines are not just for older people. Changes can begin to take place in the arteries during the teens.

Finding out:
*Your pulse rate and exercise.

Find your pulse as shown in the diagram. Take it.
Exercise strongly for two minutes then take it again. Take it after five minutes exercise.
Write down the results, perhaps in the form of a graph.

*Not to be done if you have a breathing or heart condition.

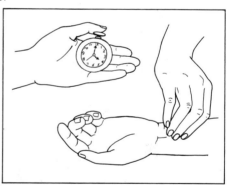

Questions

1 **Why are the infectious diseases no longer the top killers?**
2 **Name four of today's top killers. For what proportion of deaths is heart disease responsible?**
3 **Give the correct names for (a) heart muscle, (b) the tubes which carry blood.**
4 **What is blood pressure? Give the normal pulse rate of (a) an adult, (b) a toddler, (c) an adolescent.**
5 **Copy out the self-help list. Try to learn it.**

About cancer

Cancer is not one disease. It is the name for a group of diseases. Usually, there is a clump of cells, a **tumour**, which acts like a cuckoo in the nest, crowding out healthy cells, robbing them of food and oxygen, taking over and spreading to other cells nearby. It is the person's own cells which act like this – the reasons why are not properly understood.

Research into cancer

Cancer frightens some people. It is easy to understand why. Smallpox used to frighten people in much the same way until the cause of the disease was known and there was immunization against it. Now smallpox is wiped out. Research into cancer is enormous and there is bound to be a breakthrough – much is already known. The most important fact is that many cancers can be treated and cured *if they are found early enough.*

The causes

As far back as 1775, soot was found to cause cancer in chimney-sweeps. Later, people working with X-rays developed cancer of the skin. It is thought about eighty per cent of all cancers are caused by things which *irritate* the cells in some way. Anything which does this is called a **carcinogen**. There is now a long list of carcinogens – tar, asbestos, chromium, tobacco smoke, and nuclear radiation are a few. Viruses (pp. 18–19) cause cancer in animals and, probably, humans. Over-exposure to strong sunlight can cause cancer of the skin.

Cures for cancer

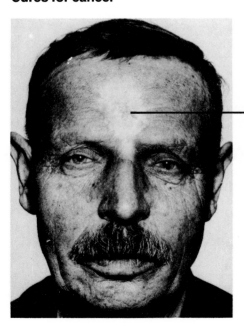

People still think there are no cures for cancer. There are. **Leukaemia** used to be a hopeless cancer of the blood in small children. Modern drugs can now cure nearly fifty per cent of all cases of leukaemia. You can see from the photograph that skin cancer can also be treated and cured. And cancer of the cervix (p. 153) can be removed with an almost one hundred per cent rate of cure – if the disease is found early enough.

Finding cancer early

Because some people are frightened of cancer, they don't go to the doctor when something is wrong. They don't want to hear bad news. But it is very bad news to let cancer cells go on spreading and growing. Many cancers can be treated and cured if they are found early enough. This is why people need to know the early warning signs. They may not be signs of cancer but they are indications that something is going wrong which needs to be checked by a doctor.

Some early warning signs

A lump in the breast, neck, armpit – anywhere.
A cough or hoarse voice lasting more than three weeks.
Difficulty in swallowing or long-lasting indigestion.
A rapid loss of weight for no obvious reason.
A sore or ulcer which doesn't heal after three weeks.
A wart or mole which turns black and begins to grow.
Bleeding on going to the lavatory; or between periods; or after the menopause (p. 123).

Self help

Most cancers take a long time to grow – these signs are for older people. But girls can examine their breasts so they can recognize changes later on.

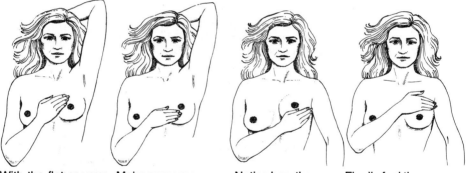

With the flat or your hand, feel the breast for any lumps.

Make sure you bring your fingers right up under the nipple.

Notice how the lower part of the breast is felt too.

Finally feel the upper, outer part. Do this lying down, perhaps in the bath.

Further information for women is given on p. 153. Both sexes should not smoke. Cancer of the mouth, the throat, and the bladder – as well as the lungs – are caused by tobacco smoke (p. 98).

Questions

1 **In your own words, explain what is meant by cancer.**
2 **Name two kinds of work which used to cause cancer.**
3 **What is a carcinogen? Name four different kinds.**
4 **Can cancer be treated and cured? Give at least two examples in your answer.**
5 **'Cancer is too horrid to think about.' Write a brief essay on why this attitude could be dangerous.**

About smoking

Of all the killer diseases which can be avoided, perhaps those caused by smoking come top of the list. Tobacco smoke is noxious (harmful), whether it comes from pipes, cigars, or cigarettes. The things which do most harm are tar, carbon monoxide, and nicotine.

1 **Tobacco tar** is an irritant, which damages the breathing tubes and lungs.
2 **Carbon monoxide** is a gas which cuts down the amount of oxygen carried in the blood. It also damages the heart and the arteries.
3 **Nicotine** is a drug which you become addicted to (hooked on). It causes over-activity of the heart and narrows both big and small arteries.

Damage

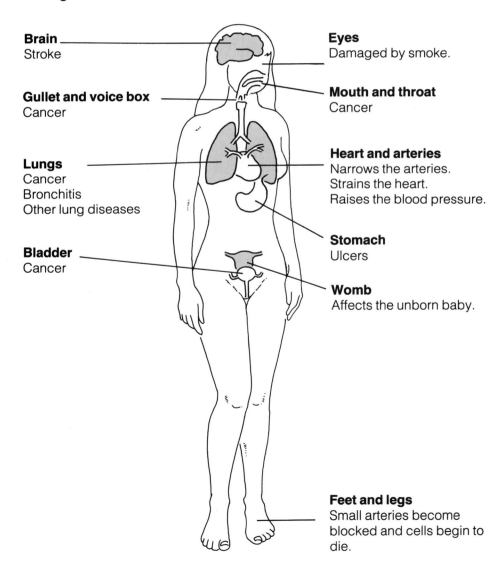

Brain
Stroke

Eyes
Damaged by smoke.

Gullet and voice box
Cancer

Mouth and throat
Cancer

Lungs
Cancer
Bronchitis
Other lung diseases

Heart and arteries
Narrows the arteries.
Strains the heart.
Raises the blood pressure.

Stomach
Ulcers

Bladder
Cancer

Womb
Affects the unborn baby.

Feet and legs
Small arteries become blocked and cells begin to die.

Health education is about staying fit and healthy, and preventing disease. It is not about morbid tales of early death from smoking. However, because smoking does so much damage to so many different parts of the body, people must know how dangerous it is. Tobacco smoke *is* a carcinogen (p. 96).

When people first inhale (breathe the smoke into their lungs), their eyes sting and water. They feel a bit dizzy, a bit queasy (sick) and slightly faint. These feelings quickly pass as the body and mind become used to the drug. There are no more warnings signs until the 'smoker's cough' begins – by which time a great deal of damage has been done.

Self help

Do not start smoking. If you already have, then stop.

Smoking is a habit. You can break any habit *if you want to enough*. But you must bring that habit back under the control of your will. Nobody can do this for you. The decision has to come from inside yourself. It is likely you have already broken certain childish habits you wanted to stop. Try to remember what helped you most then. There is a good chance those same things will help you again.

Finding out:

About tar in tobacco smoke.

Ask a smoker to exhale a few times through a clean handkerchief or a paper tissue. Examine the results.

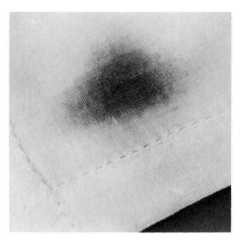

Questions

1 **In what simple way can killer diseases caused by smoking be wiped out?**
2 **Name the things in tobacco smoke which are noxious, then copy out the three points about them.**
3 **In your own words, explain the ways in which smoking can cause heart disease.**
4 **In your own words, explain the ways in which smoking can cause cancer. You may need to re-read pages 96–7.**
5 **When a person first inhales tobacco smoke, what are the signs that smoking affects the body and the mind?**
6 **A thirteen-year-old has just taken up smoking. List the ways in which you might help him or her to stop.**

More about smoking

Smoking used to be thought harmless – just a waste of money, or a fiddly habit which caused unpleasant breath. But as more and more research is done, so more and more damaging facts are discovered. Most older smokers would like to stop. But nicotine is addictive. They find it difficult to give up. They develop 'smoker's cough', which is a mixture of the sticky tar plus the extra phlegm made by the irritated breathing tubes. Smokers have more colds which last longer than non-smokers'. They develop chronic (long-term) bronchitis.

Smokers are about 14 times more likely to die from lung cancer than non-smokers are. But the chart below shows that a smoker's chances of dying from lung cancer (compared to those of a non-smoker) lessen from the time he or she gives up smoking. After about 15 years of not smoking, his or her chances of an early death are about the same as those of someone who has never smoked.

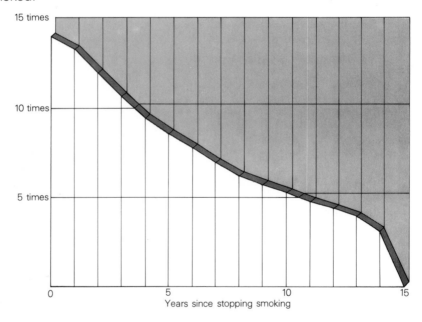

Years since stopping smoking

Passive smoking

'Passive smoking' means taking in the smoke from other people's cigarettes. Smoking has been called 'self-pollution' (making yourself dirty) but really, and sadly, it is worse than that. Because smokers pollute not only themselves but others too – usually those they love.

1 **Unborn babies** Pregnant women who smoke tend to have smaller babies than non-smokers, and their babies are more likely to be born dead or to die quite soon after birth.
2 **Children** The children of parents who smoke have more lung infections in the first years of life than the children of non-smokers.
3 **Others** Spending one hour in a smoky room can mean a non-smoker inhales the same amount of cancer-causing chemicals as a person who has smoked several filter-tip cigarettes.

A social problem

Governments put a heavy tax on pipe, cigar, and cigarette tobacco. They make a great deal of money out of smokers. However, treatment for people with diseases caused by smoking is very expensive – in Britain it costs several hundred thousand pounds a day. Also, millions of working days are lost each year because of diseases caused by smoking and smoking causes the death of over a thousand people a week. Smokers *can* stop if they *really want to* (p. 65). Anti-smoking clinics and other organizations have been set up to help.

Why do people start smoking?

Smoking usually begins in adolescence. This is why it is important that you should know all the facts. If you come from a home where parents smoke, you are likely to start. If you want to appear more 'grown-up' than you really are, you are also likely to start. But do you follow everything parents do? And is it really 'grown-up' to smoke now the dangerous facts are known?

Self help

Learn to say 'no'. Do not let people put pressure on you to start. Sadly, smoking is not something you can start and then stop. Studies have shown that a teenager who smokes just two or three cigarettes has a seventy per cent chance of becoming addicted. They also show another, quite curious, thing. The more intelligence you have – stamina, reason, self-control – the less likely you are to start.

Finding out:

The work of anti-smoking clinics.

Write or call at your local health education office. Ask for details on (a) helping addicted people to stop smoking and (b) teaching materials for use in junior schools.

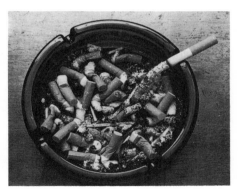

Questions

1 **Why do some older people find smoking difficult to stop?**
2 **What is a 'smoker's cough'?**
3 **Write a short essay on 'passive smoking'.**
4 **Set up a role-play scene in which a teenager refuses to join friends in smoking, then is persuaded to give in. Notice whether the words used apply to the emotions or the intelligence.**
5 **Set up the same scene. This time the teenager is able to persuade one other person to stop. Notice the same things as in the previous scene.**

About alcohol

Alcohol is a mood-changing drug. It is also **toxic** (poisonous). If you drink too much of it, you die. This does not happen often, as a drinker usually gets sick or becomes unconscious first. Alcohol slows down the working of the mind, which is why it is called a **depressant**. This can be hard to believe when you see a drunk person behaving in a wildly excited way – laughing crazily, taking dares, arguing, fighting, and smashing things up.

Why do people drink?

Usually to feel 'good', to cheer themselves up. Alcohol damps down the intelligence – the **criticizing** part of the mind. Older people have a couple of drinks to relax after work – to shrug off the tensions of the day. Younger people may be seeking excitement – they may hope to make new friends and to stop feeling self-conscious and shy. So alcohol can be useful when it helps to get rid of tension, and to cheer people up. But – and there is always a very important 'but' when it comes to any kind of drug – alcohol works in a sly and rather cruel sort of way.

Study the diagrams carefully to work out how alcohol gradually damps down the brain (1 unit = one drink – see p. 104).

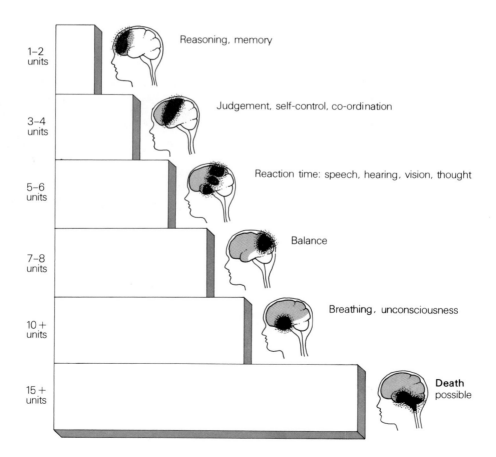

1–2 units	Reasoning, memory
3–4 units	Judgement, self-control, co-ordination
5–6 units	Reaction time: speech, hearing, vision, thought
7–8 units	Balance
10 + units	Breathing, unconsciousness
15 + units	**Death** possible

'What's your poison?'

Drinkers say this jokingly. Sadly, it is true. Alcohol is a poison, and it does kill. Look again at the diagrams. You will see that the first part of the mind to be drugged is the intelligence. This means useful things like self-control and memory, and nice things like sensitivity and insight, are quickly wiped out. The emotions are set free – there is no judgement left to hold them back. Hence the wild crazy laughter or the bitter black rage; and the dreadful things said and done – the cruel risks taken with innocent people's lives.

The trap

A little alcohol cheers people up. They talk freely, laugh happily, and are able to relax. Why should something which gives pleasure end up giving so much pain? The trap about alcohol is the order in which it works. Once you become cheerful, you cannot *remember* to stop drinking, you have no *reason* to work this out. After three or four drinks, you have lost the *self-control* to stop, you cannot *judge* that you have had too much.

'I really shouldn't. Well, just one more,' says the drinker who has lost self-control.
'I drive better when I'm drinking,' says the person whose judgement has gone.

The trap about alcohol is that drinkers do not know they have lost their intelligence *because they have lost it*! The drunker they get, the more they *feel* it is a very good idea to go on drinking!

Self help
Heavy drinkers sometimes have a false and proud image. They may sneer at the young – 'can't hold their drink'. Try not to let this taunt upset you. Having no tolerance to a drug means you are not likely to end up an alcoholic – or addicted. Practise saying 'no' very firmly. See how often you win!

Questions

1 **What is alcohol? What does 'toxic' mean?**
2 **Death from an overdose of alcohol can happen but it is rare. Give reasons why this is so.**
3 **Why is alcohol called a 'depressant'?**
4 **'Alcohol damps down the criticizing part of your mind.' Can you work out how it helps young people not to feel shy? Give reasons for your answer.**
5 **In your own words, explain the trap about alcohol.**

More about alcohol

The facts

1 After heart disease and cancer, alcohol is the third biggest health hazard today.
2 It kills, maims, and drives mentally ill more people than all the other drugs put together.
3 A third of all deaths on the road are caused by drunken drivers – many others are left hopelessly crippled or maimed (p. 114).
4 In the late evenings, violent drinkers fill up the prison cells – their victims fill up the Accident and Emergency wards in hospitals.
5 Alcohol causes **cirrhosis** (hardening) of the liver and damage to the heart and kidneys. It also shrinks the cells of the brain.
6 Like all drugs, alcohol stealthily yet steadily builds up a craving for more.
7 Alcohol is the most widely used drug and the biggest drug problem today.

Alcohol content

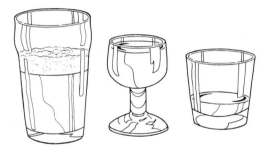

There is the same alcohol content in one half a pint of beer, one glass of wine, and one measure of spirits (whisky, gin, vodka). Each separate drink is called a *unit*. For older drinkers, six units a day are the maximum the man's body can cope with. Four units a day are the maximum for women as, on average, they weigh twenty per cent less than men. A pregnant woman should not drink more than two units a day, or she risks harming her unborn child. Young drinkers should not go above half these amounts.

Eating before you go to a party – 'lining the stomach' – does not stop you getting drunk. But it will slow down the speed at which alcohol drugs your brain.

Building up tolerance

Regular heavy drinking gets the mind 'used to' alcohol. This is called **tolerance**, and happens with nearly all drugs. Either the body or mind (or both) can tolerate the drug, and the person needs more doses and in greater strength to produce the same effects. Young people, however, have little or no tolerance. After a few drinks, they become violently sick. If they then go on drinking, they behave in odd, often dangerous, and usually highly embarrassing ways.

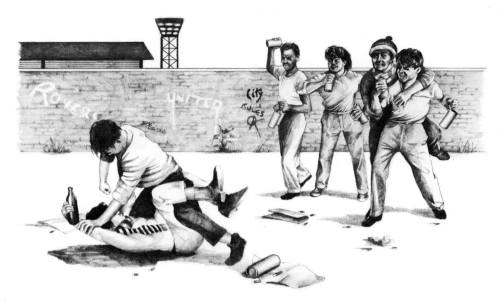

Self help

Remember the trap. You can beat it with little tricks. Only take half a bottle of wine to the party; only have enough money on you to buy two drinks. It is easy to be tempted by alcohol in the teens when you feel a bit insecure. But if you rely on alcohol to stop insecure feelings, you risk falling into a deeper trap. Can you work out what this is? (See pp. 106–7.)

Finding out:

The legal limit for drivers.

The legal limit is measured by the amount of alcohol in the blood. Ask at your police station (a) how much this limit is and (b) how the various tests are done.

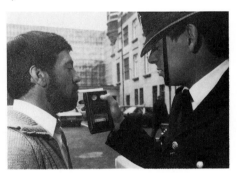

Questions

1 **From the list of facts about alcohol, choose which you think are the four worst. Copy them out and explain why you have chosen them.**
2 **What is the maximum number of units a grown man can cope with? Why can women cope with less?**
3 **In your own words, explain the ways in which young people with no tolerance to alcohol are likely to behave.**
4 **What happens when a person can tolerate a drug of any kind?**
5 **Advertisements for alcohol are subtle. Choose a few – big masterful men swilling big masterful pints; sleek sophisticated women sipping sleek sophisticated drinks. Paste them in your book and write your own comments underneath.**

About drug abuse

The use of drugs is discussed on pp. 54–5. It might be helpful now to read this unit again. The **abuse** of drugs means the perversion or misuse of them. People who abuse drugs do not suffer long-lasting diseases of the body or mind. They die, very quickly. Drug abuse is the fastest and most painful of all the kinds of damage people inflict upon themselves.

Who abuses drugs?

Young people, mainly. Older people have a great fear of drugs, especially when they read of the tragic deaths of pop stars and rock musicians who have overdosed – and drowned. Because this is how many drug addicts die. They become unconscious, they vomit, they breathe the sickness into their lungs – and drown.

The horror of drugs

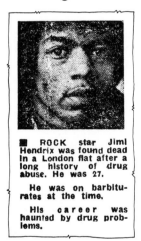

■ ROCK star Jimi Hendrix was found dead in a London flat after a long history of drug abuse. He was 27.

He was on barbiturates at the time.

His career was haunted by drug problems.

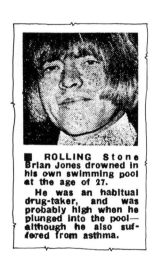

■ ROLLING Stone Brian Jones drowned in his own swimming pool at the age of 27.

He was an habitual drug-taker, and was probably high when he plunged into the pool—although he also suffered from asthma.

Compared with the numbers of young people who drink and smoke, drug taking is very rare. But because it is terrible to think of even a few young people dying in such a horrible manner, the news is broadcast everywhere – the reports are full of pity and shock. It seems dreadful that the person most at risk is the teenager or young adult who has not yet developed full mental controls. Drugs damage the mind. The young addict has no chance of growing up.

Why do a few young people start?

1 **Curiosity** 'I'll try anything once.' Yes, but would that person try driving a fast car with no brakes? Drugs are powerfully addictive. Like the car driver, the drug-taker is quickly out of control.
2 **Pleasure** 'I like having my mind blown.' Drug-takers 'go on trips', 'have highs', 'get their minds blown'. When the drug wears off, the opposite happens, they have terrible 'lows'. These are painful withdrawal symptoms.

3 **Peer pressure** (p. 120) 'They called me cissy for not trying, so I did.' Peers are your equals. Many a drug addict started by wanting to keep up with 'friends'. Pressure can be hard to resist. Perhaps it is better to make *real* friends?

4 **Self pity** 'I'm a failure. Everybody hates me. I'm going to take drugs.' Moods of insecurity and not liking yourself *will* pass. The effects of drugs are swift, and can be fatal.

Drugs and the law

It is illegal to sell, buy, be in possession of, or use drugs which have not been prescribed by a doctor. Drug **pushers** (people who sell drugs) are given long prison sentences. Society regards them as very evil as they corrupt and do terrible damage to others. People who are drug **abusers** may be fined, sent to prison or ordered to undergo treatment.

Drug abuse is a **behaviour disorder**, which means the person's emotions and intelligence are mixed up and confused. Psychiatric help is often needed before the person can be weaned off drugs.

Self help
You probably do not need any! If you are tempted, think of the horrors which lie ahead – the infections from dirty needles, the pain of injecting into collapsed veins, the squalid begging or stealing for money, the loss of personal pride – all this can lead on from trying drugs 'just for fun!'

Finding out:
If there is drug abuse in your area.

Buy or borrow a local newspaper. Study the court reports. Make notes on how the law treats drug offenders – whether they are punished or sent for treatment.

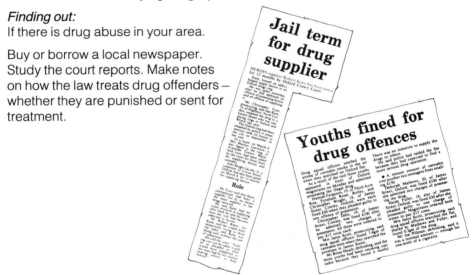

Questions

1 **What is meant by 'drug abuse'?**
2 **Who abuses drugs? Explain why the news is broadcast everywhere.**
3 **Of the four reasons why people start taking drugs, which do *you* think might be the most damaging? Give reasons for your answer.**
4 **Have a group discussion on the four reasons. Choose one and set up a role play scene in which you persuade the person not to start.**
5 **Copy out the first sentence of 'Drugs and the law'.**
6 **What is meant by a behaviour disorder?**

More about drugs (1)

Cannabis

The drug cannabis has many names – marihuana, hashish, pot, tea, ganga, and grass are a few. As cannabis has no medical use, it is not prescribed by doctors. It is imported illegally (smuggled) in very large quantities from the East, North and West Africa, India, and the West Indies. It is used in the Far East to help meditation; the assassins or Haschischiens (hashish-eaters) took it to make them ferocious; American jazz musicians believe it improves their playing and Rastafarians take it for a great variety of reasons.

The drug cannabis comes from the plant, *cannabis sativa*. Marihuana comes from the dried flowers or leaves. Hashish comes from the sticky resin and pollen. Cannabis can be made up into little cakes and eaten. More often it is smoked, sometimes mixed with tobacco leaves and rolled into a cigarette. To get the full effects of the drug, the smoke must be inhaled deep inside the lungs.

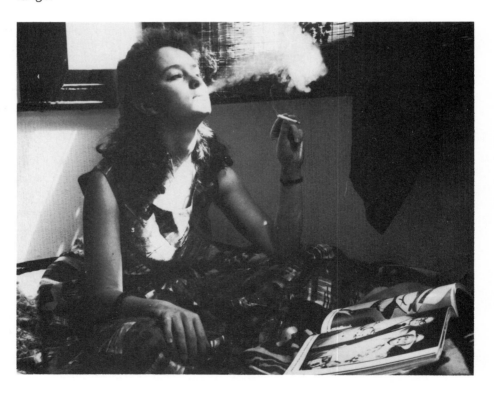

What effects does cannabis have?

The physical effects are reddening of the eyes, dilation (widening) of the pupils, an unsteady walk, a very dry mouth, a big increase in appetite, and the person gives off a strong smell of burning grass.

As with all drugs, the effects on the mind will be different for different people. At first there is a feeling of restlessness followed by great gaiety, lots of talking and laughing. Then there is euphoria – a feeling of extreme well-being. Perception (ways of looking at things) are altered – objects change size and shape, time speeds up or stands still. If the dose is large enough, the drug-taker falls into a deep sleep.

Does cannabis have bad effects?

Like all drugs, it depends upon the person's state of mind. A whisky-drinker, for example, who starts off in a bad mood is likely to end up feeling very violent indeed. It is the same with cannabis. A nervous person, for example, can find the effects alarming – it can be terrifying to believe the ground is moving under your feet. Whether the effects of cannabis bring pleasure or fear, there is always the risk of doing something dangerous when reason and judgement are drugged.

The arguments over cannabis

Cannabis is not addictive – the user does not become dependent on the drug. Some people believe the law should be changed and cannabis made legal. But the drug is a **hallucinogen** – it causes some people to see things which are not there. And a few people do become mentally dependent on the feelings of euphoria, and on the company of other drug-takers. This can lead to behaviour disorders – staying drugged as much of the time as possible, stealing to buy more supplies, clinging and 'childish' behaviour (p. 72). The mentally dependent person stops developing, and cannot get on with his or her life.

Self help
Cannabis has been discussed in great detail as many young people try it – even though it is illegal. There is then the chance they make the terrible mistake of believing other, far more dangerous, drugs can be tried – 'just for fun'. Remember too that the damage caused by long-term taking of cannabis is not yet known.

Questions

1 **Write down three other names for the drug cannabis.**
2 **How and from where is cannabis brought into the country?**
3 **Name two groups of people who take cannabis, and give their reasons.**
4 **What effects does cannabis have on the body?**
5 **Name three ways in which cannabis affects the mind.**
6 **In a paragraph, write about all the known bad effects cannabis can have.**
7 **Look up the word 'assassin'. Have a group discussion on whether a drug which makes killers ferocious is likely to be as harmless as some people think.**
8 **'The damage caused by long-term taking of cannabis is not yet known.' Write a short essay, discussing whether you think this drug should be made legal so that it can be bought and sold and used like cigarettes and alcohol.**

More about drugs (2)

The narcotics

These are the 'hard' drugs. The opiates, morphine and heroin, come from the seeds of the opium poppy. Cocaine and drugs such as dicanol are also narcotics. A narcotic is a substance which when swallowed, inhaled, or injected causes stupor, sleep, or unconsciousness depending on how much is taken. Narcotics are used medically to deaden great pain. They are called 'hard' drugs as the user quickly develops tolerance and becomes addicted.

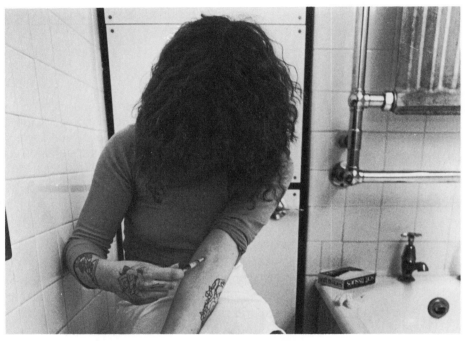

Narcotics are taken illegally by people who abuse drugs for the 'highs' – short-lived feelings of euphoria and pride. As soon as the effects wear off, the user feels extreme distress and needs another dose immediately. As the tolerance level rises, so the person becomes dreadfully ill. Many infections spread because of shared dirty hypodermic needles; veins in the arms collapse; needles are stuck anywhere – even in the groin. The narcotic addict is likely to die within a few years; from infection, suicide, or an overdose (p. 106).

The sedatives

Sedatives are used medically to reduce anxiety, and as sleeping pills. The sedative drugs are barbiturates. They work rather like alcohol. The user often seems drunk: the signs are slurred speech, a staggering walk, mental confusion, and deep sleep. Also like alcohol, tolerance to barbiturates develops rapidly. The sedative abuser is depressed and may commit suicide or take an overdose by mistake as the memory is wiped out. Alcohol taken with barbiturates kills.

The stimulants

These are amphetamines or 'pep' pills and are used medically to treat depression. The young addict may use them to stop the sleepiness from barbiturates. Both together are called 'uppers and downers'. Abusers of amphetamines end up injecting massive doses directly into a vein. This is called 'speeding'. It produces terrifying feelings which may cause a brief psychosis (p. 90).

The hallucinogens

Like cannabis, the hallucinogens are not used medically. The effects of an LSD 'trip' vary and often depend on the mood of the user. There are reports of mystical experiences; there are other reports of truly fearful or horrifying happenings. An English musician hurled himself off the roof; a Scandanavian woman stabbed her lover; a Swiss doctor jumped (from ecstasy) into a lake – and nearly drowned! Very small quantities of LSD have powerful effects and drug-takers can never be sure of what they are buying. An overdose of LSD can lead to psychosis, or death.

The solvents

These are toxic chemicals such as glue, lighter fluid, and paint thinner. Young children may sniff them for quick thrills, or 'highs'. The toxins build up in the body and can cause permanent damage. Solvent sniffing is tragic as young children die from it.

What would you do?
Fifteen-year-old Mary noticed a group of young children with chemical solvents and plastic bags. One of them was being sick. Should she go to their parents, their teachers, or the police? Would that be sneaking? Should she tell the children off herself? Would they listen to her, and stop? Or would they wait until she had gone, and then carry on?

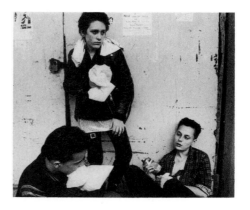

Explain what *you* would do in Mary's place.

Questions

1 **What is the definition of a narcotic drug?**
2 **Name three narcotics. What is their medical use?**
3 **What is the likely end of a heroin addict?**
4 **Explain the ways in which sedatives act rather like alcohol (p. 102).**
5 **Describe the ways in which a young addict may use stimulants.**
6 **Write a short account of the advice you would give a friend who knew nothing about LSD and wanted to take it 'just for fun'.**

Accidents and safety

In industrialized countries, accidents cause about three per cent of all deaths. The number of people injured is far higher – about five hundred for every death. Many accidents are **preventable**. This means they *could have* been avoided which, in turn, means they *should have* been avoided. Learning about health must include learning about safety. No-one wants to be the cause of a preventable accident.

The main causes of accidental death

Age group	Annual number of deaths from all causes per 100, 000 people	Percentage of deaths resulting from accidents	Chief causes of accidental death (as percentage of total)	Commonest other causes (in order of frequency)
Under 1	140	3%	Choking and suffocation (70%)	Falls; fire; road accidents
1–4	55	28%	Road accidents (37%)	Fire; drowning; choking and suffocation
5–9	30	38%	Road accidents (57%)	Drowning; fire; falls
10–14	25	37%	Road accidents (53%)	Drowning; choking and suffocation; falls
15–24	65	55%	Road accidents (76%)	Poisoning; falls; drowning
25–44	120	17%	Road accidents (53%)	Poisoning; falls; choking and suffocation
45–64	1, 000	3%	Road accidents (44%)	Falls; poisoning; fire
Over 64	6, 000	2%	Falls (61%)	Road accidents; fire; poisoning

You can see that the most dangerous place is the road – for drivers, passengers, cyclists, *and* pedestrians. The kitchen is often the most dangerous room in the house – fires usually start here, and so do terrible accidents to the very old and the young. Falls are a common cause of death, especially for the elderly. Choking and suffocation are caused by breathing into plastic bags, by swallowing unchewed lumps of food, or by inhaling vomit (p. 106). Drowning can happen when children are left unattended – in the bath, near open pools, or by the sea.

Safety first!

1 Everyone needs to remember how dangerous traffic can be. Children should be taught to fear the road by older people's example. Always obey the traffic rules.
2 The home should be made as safe as possible, especially against fire. Do not leave boxes of matches lying around, pan handles sticking out from the stove, or fires without guards. To protect against falls: stair carpets should be firmly attached, child-proof gates fixed at the top of the stairs, doors and windows securely locked, and non-slip mats used on floors.
3 Small children have to be watched. Parents and older people in the family must be aware that a child cannot remember safety rules at first. Knives, tablets, bottles of bleach, trailing electric wires, the cooker are all things which fascinate a child. You have to be the 'eyes and the ears' – you are the person who prevents accidents happening to the child.

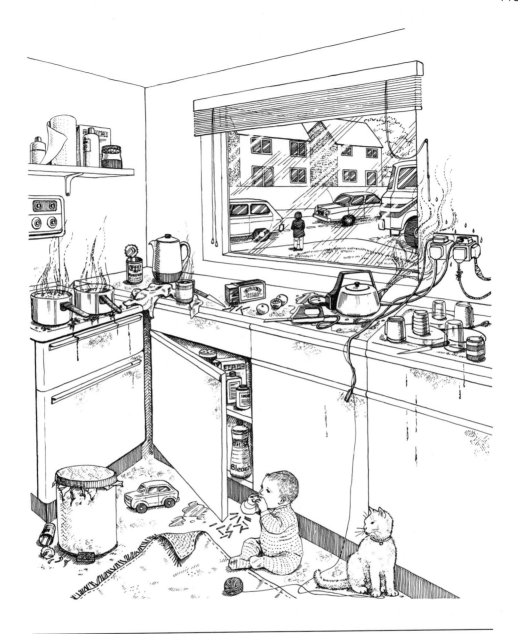

Questions

1 **What is meant by a 'preventable' accident? And why does learning about health include learning about safety?**

2 **Nowadays, babies are often put on their stomachs to sleep. From the chart, write down why you think this is so.**

3 **What age groups are most likely to die from drowning? Give reasons why you think this is so, and what safety precautions should be taken.**

4 **Study carefully the picture above. Make as long a list as you can of all the possible dangers. Beside each point, write down what should be done to avoid the accident.**

Adolescent safety

'If only – '

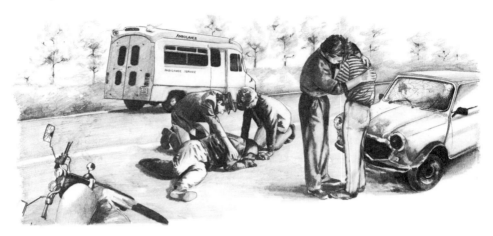

These must be amongst the saddest words ever. 'If *only* I hadn't dared him.' 'If *only* she'd been watching out.' Deaths from accidents are the single biggest killer of people between the ages of fifteen and twenty-four. You can see from the chart on page 112 that over three-quarters of these deaths happen on the road. And many more young people suffer *spinal injuries* which make them physically disabled – or *head injuries* which can cause mental handicap (p. 156). Road Traffic Accidents are called RTAs by police, by ambulance drivers, and by hospital staff.

Why are there so many RTAs?

High spirits, lack of concentration, taking risks – these are partly the reasons why teenagers dash out into the road. But far too many RTAs are caused by young people drinking and driving – it is hard to believe they do not know how dangerous alcohol is (p. 104). Even among people who never drink, the number of young men drivers involved in RTAs is very high indeed. If you drive, especially if you drive a motor-bike, you must take extra special care.

1 Keep your bike or car in really good roadworthy condition.
2 Regularly check your brakes, steering, lights, tyres, and mirrors.
3 Know the Highway Code and all the safety precautions by heart.
4 Regard other road users as potentially lethal – their mistake could be your death.
5 Make sure your own driving is faultless – always!

Other causes of accidents

If you look back to the chart, you will notice the word 'poisoning'. After RTAs, poisoning is the next most common cause of death among people between fifteen and forty-four. But poisoning from what? Have you already guessed? Drug overdose, which is nearly always accidental. Often large amounts of alcohol are also found in the blood.

Thrills and spills

Part of being a teenager is the need to experiment, and to test yourself out. Taking dares to do something wildly dangerous, drinking alcohol, or trying drugs – these can be seen as terrifically thrilling things to do. But drugs kill, and those people who don't die in 'drink and drive' accidents can end up crippled for life.

Danger is thrilling, yes; especially when you are young. But you need to find a way to get thrills and spills without damaging your life. Find a sport which suits *your* needs for excitement – hill climbing, ice-skating, football, whatever suits *you*. Where is the thrill, after all, in ending up dead!

Self help

Are you accident-prone? Some people do seem to have more minor accidents than others. They drop things, bump into things – they are all bruises and cuts. If this is happening to you, it could be you have not yet adjusted to your changing body shape (p. 12). However, there is a chance you could be acting too impulsively (p. 72). If you keep having minor accidents, then this is not behaviour which suits you right now. Slow down and concentrate on your movements for a little while. You will find you can speed up again quite soon – if you want to.

Finding out:
About the Highway Code

Borrow a copy from the library – it is written for pedestrians as well as drivers. Choose a section which interests you and do a full project on it.

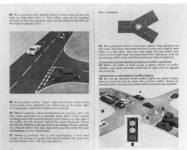

Preventable accidents

The word 'accident' is often used to mean chance or bad luck. Yet almost all accidents are caused by human error – the mistakes people make. This whole section has been very solemn, and full of the most gruesome health hazards. But it is *your* mind and *your* body, and you are the person responsible for them. You are free to make your own health choices, just like everyone else.

Questions

1 **Write a short essay, which ends with the words 'If only I had taken more care.'**
2 **Make a list of all the reasons you can think of why drivers should not race one another on a public highway.**
3 **Write about the second most common cause of death among young people.**
4 **Do you agree that teenagers need to test themselves and to experiment? Give reasons for your answer.**
5 **Do you think people should be free to make their own health choices? Have a discussion about this.**

Further work on Chapter 3

1 Changes can begin to take place in the arteries during the teens. Write an essay, describing how to guard against heart disease.

2 An older person passes blood when going to the lavatory. He says nothing, hoping it will stop. What advice does he need, and why?

3 Find out about the effects of nuclear radiation. Ask at your library for information on the outbreak of leukaemia among Japanese survivors of the atomic bomb.

4 Find out how much tax is on one packet of cigarettes. Then find out how much revenue your government gets from smokers each year. A few people call this 'dirty' money – they are usually smokers. Would you increase the tax or change it in any way? Give reasons for your answer.

5 Collect some of the sillier advertisements for cigarettes – the great outdoor life; pure gold; the smart life-style. Have a discussion on whether they appeal to the emotions (dreams, fantasies) or the intelligence. Write what you think might be more suitable copy.

6 From your local police station, find out the numbers of road accidents caused by drunken driving last year.

7 'Alcohol is like fire. It makes a good servant but a punishing master.' Write a short essay, discussing this statement.

8 Visit or write to your local Alcoholics Anonymous office. Ask for details about (a) the help they give to the addicted person and (b) the advice they give to their families.

9 Do you think drug-taking is emotional or intelligent behaviour? Try to give as many reasons as you can for your answer.

10 'The fault is not in the drug, but in the person.' Write a short essay, discussing whether you agree with this statement or not.

11 Most narcotic addicts take drugs to give themselves a sense of well-being. Turn to page 60 and re-read the three things this includes. Taking each point separately, write about whether you think addicts achieve a sense of well-being or not.

12 Falls are the chief cause of accidental death in the elderly. List at least three safety measures you would take to prevent falls in the home.

13 Give four causes of fire in the home. In each example, say how safety awareness can prevent fire.

14 Write about a time when you were responsible for an accident which could have been prevented. How did you feel? Did you learn anything from the experience?

15 Young people often have to pay a higher premium for insurance against driving accidents. Give all the reasons why you think this is so.

16 'Nearly all accidents are caused by human error.' Do you agree, or disagree? Give as many examples as you can to explain your answer.

17 You have a friend who lives on chips, beer, cigarettes, and nervous tension. Explain all the risks your friend is taking wth the top killers.

Chapter 4

About relationships

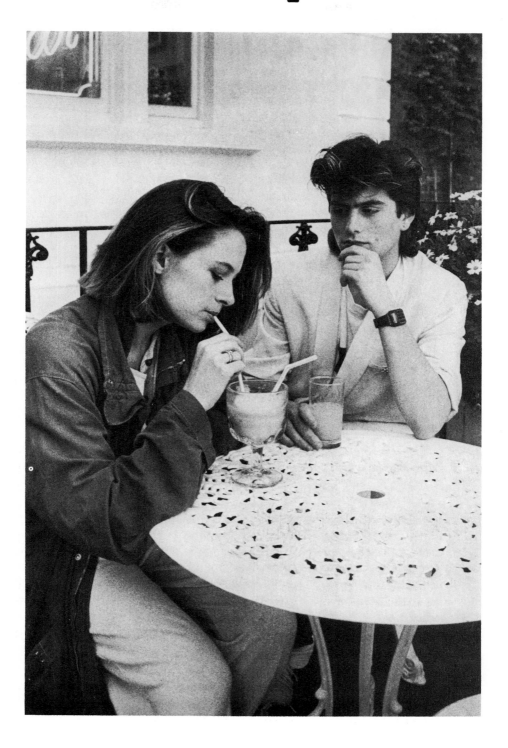

About conflicts with adults

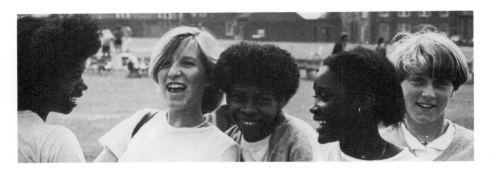

'I want my future to start now. Like yesterday.'
'I'm in no hurry. Being my age is really great.'
'I can't decide. One day I'm grown up, the next day I feel a kid.'

Some people start their future early – by 18 they are married with a couple of children. Others start slowly – 28, they decide, is soon enough to settle down. While others just drift along, letting things happen and not making plans. People are different and what suits one person may not suit another. But can you guess which of the people quoted above might be in conflict with adults? And why?

The 'make or break' years

The teens are a very important time. They are the 'make or break' years for your future. Decisions you take now will almost certainly affect the rest of your life. Adults know this and try to help you towards the 'best' decisions. Often this means giving you advice about not starting your future too early, or leaving it too late. Most teenage conflicts with adults centre around this timing. Are they right? Or are you?

How can you tell?

If you watch small children having tea, you will notice certain things. Usually, they cannot wait till everyone is served, they begin eating at once. They quickly lose interest in the food and ask what is coming next. If the food is difficult to chew, they are likely to spit it out. They cannot choose between two cakes, they cannot bear the responsibility of making the wrong choice. They may snatch at the food on someone else's plate immediately after giving that person a kiss.

This is natural behaviour for a small child (p. 72). But would you think it reasonable if an adult acted like this? Study the chart and match the child's behaviour at tea with each of the different points.

Child	Adult
wants things at once	can put off pleasure now for future rewards
likes lots of change	can stick patiently at one project
avoids difficult work	can work diligently at unpleasant tasks
is afraid of choice	can accept responsibility for choice of actions
has shallow sympathy	can give deep sympathy and positive help

Of course not all grown-ups do these things, and not all children are so demanding. But the adult *mind* is capable of them, whereas the child's mind is not. If you are unlucky enough to be in conflict with adults, study the chart again. It is natural that your behaviour in the teens will swing between the two sides. But are you using your *intelligence* over your conflicts?

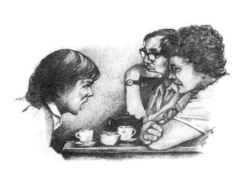 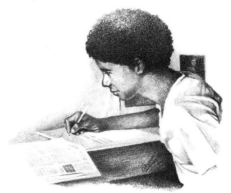

At 15, Zoe rebels against her parents. She screams that she hates them and wants to punish them. Her mother weeps. Her father storms. Zoe does not care. She truants from school, takes up smoking and drinking, then is caught stealing from a shop and has to appear in a Juvenile Court.

At 15 too, Zack rebels against his parents. He says nothing. He works extra hard at school, refuses to join a gang (p. 120), and applies for a job abroad. Later when the job falls through, Zack is secretly pleased. He has passed the rebelling stage and would hate to be so far from home.

People, whatever their age, tend to take out their bad feelings on those nearest to them. In the teens, it is parents who usually get attacked. Zack did not make this mistake, though he did plan to get away. Later, there were no wounds from hurt feelings which needed to be patched up.

Points to discuss

1 The longing to be free and independent can be so powerful in the teens that some people become too impatient and risk losing sight of their goals (p. 84).
2 Some adults are far from perfect and deserve the attacks they get.

Questions

1 **What would you consider a 'wrong' decision in the 'make or break' years of the teens? Explain how it would affect that person's whole future.**
2 **Do you agree, or disagree, that most conflicts with adults are about the teenager's future? Give reasons for your answer.**
3 **Copy out the Child/Adult chart. In what ways does it show that children behave emotionally (impulsively), and adults can behave intelligently (p. 72)?**
4 **Have a discussion about Zoe and Zack's behaviour. Who else do you think Zoe is punishing, apart from her parents? What advice would you give her?**
5 **Try to match first Zoe's, and then Zack's, behaviour against the points on the Child/Adult chart.**

Adolescent peer groups

Peer groups

Your 'peers' are your 'equals'. A peer group is the name for people of about the same age, background, and interests. During the teens, peer group friendships are very popular. There may be up to ten people in any one group. Adults sometimes worry about peer groups; they worry about their children 'getting in with the wrong set'. Here are some facts on groups you might like to discuss.

Friendship groups

Members share the same **values** (ways of looking at life), have similar interests, and are close companions. They are usually all the same sex. They do not allow people who are very 'different' to join the group. There is no leader. Each person has an equal standing in the group.

Gangs

A gang has a leader who lays down the rules. There is a strict **hierarchy** – each member has a higher or lower place in the group and must stay in it. Gangs are usually single sex, more often boys than girls. Loyalty to the gang can be more important than sharing values or making close friends.

Peer group pressure

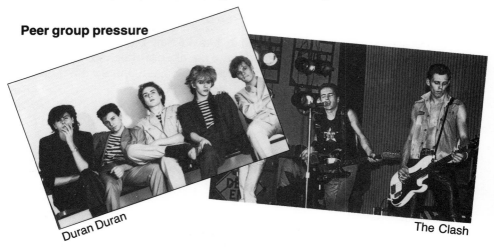

Duran Duran

The Clash

The need to **conform** (to be the same as your peers) is quite strong in the teens. At the same time, there is a need to be different from the rest of society, *and* to be different from other groups. Fashions in dress, music, and behaviour are chosen to show the values of the group. These values range from wanting to look, sound, and be unattractive to wanting to appear smart and sophisticated, or romantic and very attractive.

A group also shows the values it holds by the behaviour it chooses. Each member of the group is expected to conform to this behaviour. This is called **peer group pressure**. It is very difficult to hold out against. In fact, it can be almost impossible to 'belong' and *not* be swayed by the values of the group.

The dangers

Some teenagers have a confused self-image – they do not yet know who they really are. People in this state can be swallowed up by *the values* of the group. They may believe everything they are told. They can lose their judgement and their common sense.

Deviant behaviour
Deviant means turning aside, swerving off the track. Deviant behaviour in groups includes fighting and breaking the law. Perfectly nice people who would never be deviant on their own can be swayed by the pressure of the group. It is easy to be 'brave' in numbers. Cowards roam the streets, 'bravely' beating up the helpless, the weak, and the old.

Getting stuck
On a much milder level, people who let the group swallow them whole are slow to develop a clear self-image. They risk getting stuck at the confused, uncertain stage. This is because it is difficult to move forward without adult company. You can only learn **parallel** (side-by-side) experiences from your peers. You can only swop similar teenage happenings.

But in adult company, you can learn how adults tackle problems, how adults make decisions, the sort of situations adults try to avoid, and so on. This kind of learning helps you develop a clearer image of yourself, and a clearer idea of how *you* will behave in the adult world.

Self help
1 Find out the values of a group before you join. Always keep a small part of yourself separate so there is no risk of you being swallowed up.
2 A good way to find suitable friends is to join a club or go to evening classes which deal with your own special interests.
3 Leave a group if you find their values clash with yours. This may be painful, but it is better than conforming to values you think are wrong.
4 Groups can be fun but it is not wise to cut out adult company completely.
5 Some people never join groups. They feel more comfortable on their own. The need to belong to a group fades in the late teens as relationships with the other sex become important.

Questions

1 **Which do you think more democratic (equal) – a friendship group or a gang? Give as many reasons as you can for your answer.**
2 **Do you agree a group shows its values by the fashions it chooses? Select one popular musical group and write about its image.**
3 **What is meant by 'parallel' experience? Write a short essay, explaining what you would say to help a person who had been swallowed up by the group.**
4 **'It is easy to be "brave" in numbers.' Have a discussion on this.**
5 **Do you agree or disagree with Self-help point 3? Answer this question from what you have learned about mental health and having a sense of well-being.**

About female sexual development

On pages 12–13 you read about the changes in your body shape at puberty. I may be helpful now to go back and read these pages again. The hormones which control your sexual or reproductive development are **oestrogen** and **progesterone**. These are made in the two **ovaries** – find their position in the diagram.

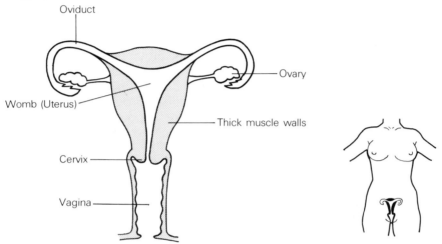

Oviduct

Ovary

Womb (Uterus)

Thick muscle walls

Cervix

Vagina

Eggs are the female reproductive (sex) cells. They ripen in the ovaries, usually one egg each month. The ripened egg travels along the **oviduct** (egg-tube) to the womb – this takes about five days. The **womb** is sometimes called the uterus. It is about the size of the girl's fist and has strong walls of muscle with a soft lining inside. When the egg reaches the womb, the lining is thick with nourishing blood in case a 'baby' is on the way.

Menstruation

This is usually called a **period**. It is monthly bleeding from the womb. When no 'baby' is on the way, the thick lining breaks down and is shed. It passes through the **cervix**, which is a ring of muscles to keep the 'baby' safely in. The period blood then flows down the **vagina**, a stretchy tube which connects the womb to the outside for the man's penis and the passage for birth. The vagina makes lubricating creams which keep its walls smooth and clean. No other hygiene is needed.

The vulva

The entrance to the vagina is protected by padded folds of skin. In front of the vagina is the opening for urine and in front of that is the **clitoris**. This is a small sensitive lump which gives great pleasure during sexual intercourse (love-making). All this area is called the **vulva**, and is covered on the outside by pubic hair. Hygiene of the vulva is very important, especially during a period.

The monthly cycle

This is counted as 28 days, but it can be any time from 23 to 35 days. Counting starts from the first day of the period – the egg is released in the middle of the month. The cycle is like this:

The womb		The ovary
Day 1	Bleeding begins.	Egg starts to ripen.
Day 5	Bleeding ends.	Egg is still ripening.
Day 14	Lining is thicker.	Egg is released into oviduct.
Day 21	Lining is ready for the 'baby'.	Egg travels to the womb.
Day 28	Unused lining is broken down.	New egg starts to ripen.

Pre-menstrual tension (PMT)

Just before a period, a few women feel rather tense. They may have slightly sore breasts, mild headaches, and a general feeling of being 'out of sorts'. This is thought to be caused by the changing amounts of hormones which control the monthly cycle. The discomfort stops as soon as bleeding begins. PMT is rare before the late teens or early twenties.

Period pains

These are 'cramps' felt when the lining of the womb breaks down. Only a third of girls have period pains, and usually they are mild. But a few unlucky people really do suffer. They need to take two aspirins and lie down. If you are one of them, do lots of exercises in between periods to tone up the whole stomach area. These exercises also tone up the muscles of the womb and this should cut down on the cramps.

A woman's fertile life

To be **fertile** is to be able to start a child. A woman's fertile life begins when her first egg is released and ends at the **menopause** (the change of life). A baby girl is born with unripened eggs already in her ovaries. Early pregnancy 13+ is not wise as the egg may not be fully ripe and there may be something wrong with the baby. Nor is late pregnancy 40+ always safe as there is a chance the egg itself is too old and the baby may have some disability.

At the menopause, no more eggs are ripened or released. Periods stop and less of the female sex hormones are produced. The average age for the menopause is now between 48 and 52, but it can happen earlier or later. Some women look forward to the end of their fertile life as it means they do not have to use birth control any more.

Questions

1 **Copy the labelled diagram of the female reproductive organs into your book, and try to learn the names of the different parts.**
2 **Name the two female hormones and say what they do.**
3 **In your own words, describe the monthly cycle from Day 1 to Day 28.**
4 **For how long in a woman's life is she fertile?**
5 **Explain what happens at the menopause.**

About male sexual development

The testicles

These are two balls which hang outside the body in a loose pouch of skin. The testicles do not hang evenly – one is usually higher than the other. They are sensitive: in times of excitement or cold weather they shrink back up against the body. Their work is to make the male sex hormone **testosterone**, and to make **sperms**.

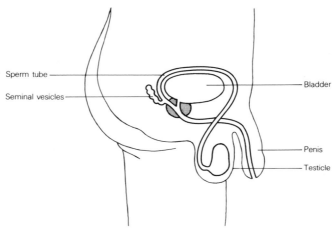

Sperms

These are the male reproductive (sex) cells. From puberty onwards, millions of sperms are constantly made. In the diagram, follow the path of sperms up the **sperm tubes**. Notice the **seminal vesicles** which pour a nourishing liquid on them. This is called **semen** – it can have up to 200 million sperms in it. Semen is pumped out of the body through the **penis**.

The penis

The penis hangs down outside the body in front of the testicles. It is soft and limp, with sponge-like spaces inside. During sexual excitement, these spaces fill up with blood fluids. The penis gets bigger and firm, and stands away from the body. This is called an **erection**. Without an erection, the penis cannot enter the woman's vagina.

The top of the penis is called the **glans**. It is very sensitive and gives great pleasure during sexual intercourse. The glans is protected by the **foreskin**, which can easily slide back. A lubricating cream, **smegma**, is made under the foreskin to keep the glans smooth and clean.

Circumcision

In circumcision, the foreskin is pushed back from the glans and cut off. About one-sixth of all males are circumcised as a religious rite. This happens to

Jewish boys soon after birth and to Moslem boys before their teens. (A few Moslem girls also have the inner folds of the vulva cut.) Other parents have their baby boys circumcised from custom – it used to be the normal practice.

If the foreskin is too tight, it is difficult to pass water or to have erections. But this is *very* rare, and circumcision is now considered quite unnecessary. However, uncircumcised males must take great care with their hygiene. If the smegma is not removed by regular washing, it gets trapped and turns stale. This makes an excellent breeding ground for germs, and the glans quickly becomes infected. Make sure you clean under the foreskin whenever you wash yourself.

Emissions

An emission means a 'sending forth'. It is the word used for when a man 'comes' – when semen is pumped out of the penis. Nocturnal means 'by night' so a **nocturnal emission** is the name for a 'wet dream' – an emission which happens during sleep. **Masturbation** is rubbing the penis, which also produces an emission. Girls masturbate too, they rub the vulva by hand.

The sex drive

This is a primitive urge to **reproduce**. It is nature's way of making sure babies continue to be born. But the sex drive can begin long before people are ready to fall in love, marry, and settle down. In fact, the sex drive has little to do with love when it first starts. This is especially true for boys, who can have erections and emissions whether they want them or not.

Masturbation and wet dreams are ways of coping with sexual tension. Both are harmless, and give pleasure. Neither are essential. For boys, sperms which are not emitted are broken down and re-used in the body. How each person, whether boy or girl, copes with sexual tension is a matter of personal and private choice.

A man's fertile life

From puberty till old age, millions of sperms are constantly being made. This means a man is fertile from the early teens till late in life. However, the sperms are not so healthy in older men and there is a chance the baby may have some disability. Can you work out the difference between a man's and a woman's fertile life?

Questions

1 **Copy the labelled diagram of the male reproductive organs into your book, and try to learn the names of the different parts.**
2 **Name the two kinds of work done in the testicles.**
3 **In your own words, say why a man's sexual hygiene is very important.**
4 **What is an emission? How many sperms can there be in one emission?**
5 **For how long in a man's life is he fertile?**

About sexual feelings

Your **fantasies** are your imaginings – the *unreal* scenes you make up in your head. From the teens onwards, people have different sexual fantasies. Here are two which are usual when sexual feelings first begin.

A girl may fantasize she is swept off her feet by some wonderful man. She is helpless to defend herself, but he is tender and kind. He makes perfect love to her. He adores her madly.

A boy may fantasize he is with a beautiful temptress – a woman who knows how to seduce a young man. He is at the mercy of her charms. She makes perfect love to him. She turns him into a man.

Responsibilities

Can you work out what these fantasies have in common? The responsibility was on the other person, not on the girl or boy. In *real* life, things are very different. People *are* responsible for what they do. Moral attitudes towards sex *are* very important indeed. The sexual act without love and responsible feelings can cause great damage.

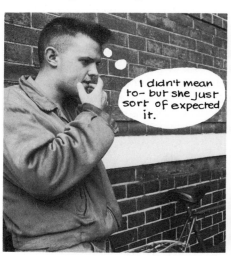
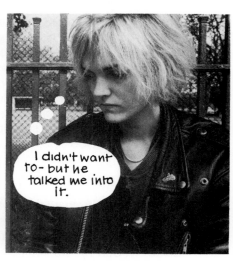

There are natural anxieties too – starting a baby, disease, fear of a broken heart, not wanting to be used, not wanting to appear clumsy, and so on. Everyone has them. Do you think it surprising that sexual fantasies are about not having any responsibility? Discuss what these two people are saying. Are they being honest about their feelings, or not?

Differences

When sexual feelings start, they can cause a few worries. Some people have powerful fantasies, others hardly think of sex at all.

'Am I "different" because I prefer study/sport to thinking about sex?'
'Am I "different" because I think of sex practically the whole time?'

Of course not. But you *are* different because you are *you*. There is no reason to expect your sexual thoughts and feelings to be the same as other people's. The sex drive is often talked of as a 'thing' on its own. It is not. It is closely bound up with the whole of you as a person.

There is another difference, too. Re-read the fantasies. A girl's are more likely to be bound up with her emotions. This may be due to secret pressures from her intelligence about the risks she is taking – not all methods of birth control work (p. 134). Unlike the boy, she may lose the chance of a career, or face the painful decision of termination of pregnancy (p. 138). Over 3,500 schoolgirls aged 15 or under become pregnant each year and another 8,500 are pregnant by the age of 16.

A boy has emotional needs too. But the pressures he is under from his erections and emissions may turn his thoughts more towards sex. However, a boy's sexual feelings depend, to a large extent, on his confidence about himself – and about women. The more thoughtful and caring he is, the more likely he is to need time to sort these things out.

Coping with pressures

Girls and boys are thought to have the same sexual feelings. But they are under different pressures to behave in different ways. Some people believe that these pressures come from 'outside' – from the society we live in. Others strongly disagree. What is your opinion? Whatever you decide, you can see that sexual feelings are not as simple as people sometimes think.

Because you have sexual feelings does not mean you have to put them into practice. *Never* give in to pressures which you think might do you harm. As well as sexual feelings, adolescence is about the development of the intelligence and the emotions too (p. 72). Early sexual activity can damage people's futures – failed exams, lost chances, broken hearts, or loveless marriages are just a few of the results. The general advice is: accept sexual feelings as a nice normal part of the teens, and wait until you are ready to give your heart and mind as well (p. 131).

Points to consider
1 Sexual feelings are as sensitive and loving as the person they belong to.
2 Many people regard sex without love or responsibility as dangerous and wrong.

Questions
1 **Love-making between happy couples is a magic, joyous thing. Yet this unit is full of warnings. Do you think them important, or not? Try to work out your answers from the mental as well as the physical health point of view.**
2 **It is unlawful to have sexual intercourse under a certain age. Find out what this age is and give reasons why you (a) agree or (b) disagree with it.**
3 **Promiscuity is the deliberate choice of having as many sexual partners as possible. Do you consider this 'good' or 'bad'?**
4 **Pornography is the obscene study – usually of women – as sex objects to be used for pleasure and nothing else. Have a discussion on this.**

About loving relationships

Crushes

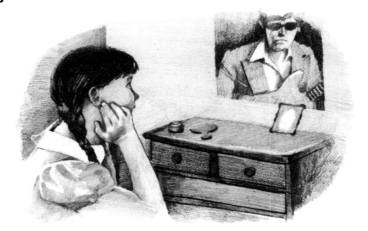

These can be thought of as a 'practice run' for later on. Crushes may be on pop stars, sports people, teachers – any person who is older and has qualities which are admired. Crushes feel like real love – they can be just as painful and just as exciting. But the difference is that the **beloved** (the love object) is admired and imitated *from a distance*. There is no real relationship. Love only travels one way.

Crushes are quite usual in the teens. They rarely last into adult life. They can be a useful way of learning how powerful and puzzling human emotions often are. The general advice is: try not to lose *too* much time on day-dreams which are unlikely to come true!

Homosexual friends

Homosexual means 'of the same sex'. **Heterosexual** means 'of the other sex'. Close friends of the same sex are perfectly natural in the teens – as at any other time. But during adolescence, the emotions can be a bit unsteady. There may be secret worries about wanting to be physically close. The general advice is: try to avoid physical contact of a sexual kind during the teens.

This is not to say that homosexual love between adults is 'bad' or 'good'. People have different opinions – everyone makes up their own mind. But homosexuals have special difficulties. Many people do not approve of them and cruel jokes are often made at their expense. Also, there can be an underlying sadness in homosexual relationships as there is no chance that children can be born from their love.

Romantic love

Romantic love is bitter-sweet: agony and ecstasy at the same time. During the bitter times, something important happens. Lovers begin to see each other as *real* people, and not just fantasies from dreams. They learn the quirky bits, the bits which don't quite match, the bits which can be slightly irritating – they learn the *un*romantic sides of love.

Courtship

As every person is different, so every loving relationship is also different. There can be no hard and fast rules about how lovers should behave. What works well for one couple may be quite wrong for another. Each loving relationship has to be specially built to suit the people in it.

Courtship is the time when lovers find out more about themselves. They have the important task of deciding whether they are right for each other, or not. Marriage today is based on love and **compatability** (being well-suited or well-matched). Adolescents often do not understand their own needs. So it is difficult for them to understand the needs of the beloved. The general advice is: try to put off serious courting until you know more about yourself.

Why is courtship important?

No one person can fulfil all your secret dreams. There will always be differences, even between the most loving couple. It takes time to learn these differences. It takes time to decide whether they matter, or not. During courting, romantic love has a chance to move a stage forward. People find they can love a *real* person, faults and all. It is very important this happens. Lovers don't want to find out they are not right for each other *after* the wedding.

Finding out:
What *you* think Belinda should do.

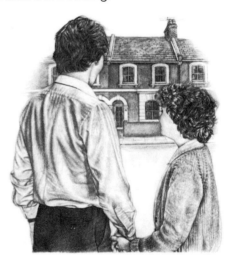

Belinda and Gavin plan to marry soon. They have put a deposit on their new home. But Belinda has secret worries. She thinks she still loves Gavin but there are sides of his character she really dislikes. She wants to break off the engagement for a while, but she doesn't want to hurt Gavin. Both sets of parents approve of the match, and she is afraid of upsetting them too.

Questions

1 **In your own words, explain why a 'crush' is not real love.**
2 **What do (a) 'homosexual' and (b) 'heterosexual' mean?**
3 **People have marvellous dreams about their beloved. What things can be learned during the 'bitter' times of romantic love? Do you think this is important? Give reasons for your answer.**
4 **What is meant by 'compatibility'? Do you think it is important? Write a story about how Belinda tries to change Gavin *after* the wedding, and with what likely results.**
5 **Do you agree or disagree with the general advice given for courtship? Explain why. What further advice do you think might be helpful?**

Love and marriage

Marriage today

Marriage today is seen as an equal relationship between the two people based on love and compatibility. This relationship includes:

1   An equal sharing of the work and the responsibilities.
2   Mutual support in times of trouble and distress.
3   The satisfaction of the sexual needs of the couple.
4   Tender loving care by both parents in the upbringing of children.
5   The provision of a secure stable home for all members of the family.
6   Personal freedom *within* the vows of marriage.
7   An equal sharing of the decisions for the good of the family.

But people don't always marry because they are madly in love. Study this list.

Wanting security
Wanting to get away from parents
Wanting a home of their own
Wanting to be like everyone else

Wanting children
Wanting someone there for company
Wanting someone to look after them
Wanting . . . just wanting to be married.

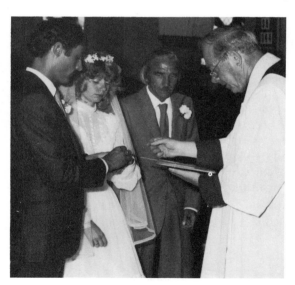

'Before you are joined in matrimony, I have to remind you of the solemn and binding character of the vows you are about to make.
Marriage is the union of one man and one woman voluntarily entered into for life to the exclusion of all others.'

Love-making

Love-making before marriage used to be forbidden. Attitudes have changed, but a recent study found that many people want to 'keep themselves' for that one special person whom they love. It is damaging to bully or persuade anyone to go against such deeply-important views. Love-making is about *sharing* – bodies, hearts, *and* minds.

Love-making is rarely perfect at the beginning; nor is it likely to be perfect every single time. The man has to learn control, to slow down and take his time. The woman has to be free of the fear of pregnancy, if the couple are not ready to start a family. The general advice is: think of *giving* pleasure rather than *getting* it. Love needs to travel both ways.

Present-day attitudes to marriage

(Totals in both tables exceed 100 per cent because more than one answer could be given.)

What do you think tends to make for a happy marriage? *(Figures are percentages)*

	Total	Men	Women
Comradeship, doing things together	29	27	30
Give-and-take, consideration	28	24	31
Discussing things, understanding	28	26	30
Mutual trust, mutual help, no secrets	20	21	19
Love, affection	19	20	18
Children	14	17	11
Shared interests	13	13	14
Sexual compatibility	5	7	3
Financial security – no debts	5	7	4
Happy home life	5	7	3
Good temper, humour	4	3	4
Home of one's own	1	1	0

What do you think tends to wreck a marriage? *(Figures are percentages)*

	Total	Men	Women
Neglect, bad communication, spouse going out	30	26	33
Selfishness, no give-and-take, intolerance	25	25	25
Infidelity, jealousy	25	29	22
Poverty, extravagance, money disagreements, wives working	17	15	19
Conflicting personalities, no common interests	12	13	12
Temper, arguing, quarrelling, fighting	10	11	9
Sexual incompatibility, fear of more children, no children	10	11	9
Lack of affection, love, general irritation	7	7	8
Drunkenness	7	7	7
Lack of trust, untruthfulness	6	6	7
No house of one's own, bad management, in-laws	4	5	4

Points to consider

1 Marriage today is seen as an equal relationship between a man and a woman.
2 People expect a great deal of personal happiness from the married state.
3 One in three marriages break down (a) when people marry under 20; (b) when there is a baby already on the way.
4 The older the couple when they marry, the more chance there is of the marriage being a success.
5 Marriage does not suit everyone. There is nothing 'bad' or 'good' about choosing to live alone.

Questions

1 **Copy out the seven points under 'Marriage today'. Do you agree with them, or not? Give reasons for your answer.**
2 **What other points do you think could be added to the list? Have a discussion before answering this.**
3 **People don't always marry because they are madly in love. From the list, choose those reasons which you think might (a) help or (b) hinder a marriage, and say why.**
4 **Study the chart carefully before filling in your own responses.**

Family planning

Family planning helps a couple control their fertility. They can choose how many children they wish to have, and when to have them. The most fertile time for both sexes is in the mid-20s: see pages 123 and 125 for the different lengths of fertile life.

If a couple marry at 22 and want two children, they will need family planning for many years. There are different methods to choose from, so couples can decide which one suits them best. It is likely throughout a couple's fertile life they will vary the family planning method they use from time to time.

How human life begins

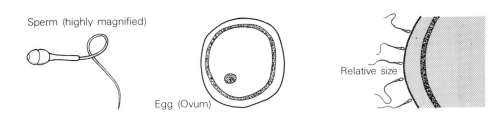

Sperm (highly magnified)

Egg (Ovum)

Relative size

After love-making, millions of sperms from the man's penis are left inside the woman's vagina. They swim through the tiny opening of the cervix, up through the womb and out into one of the oviducts. They crowd around the egg until one sperm manages to break in. The walls of the egg harden and no more sperm can get in. The sperm and the egg fuse together to become *one* new cell, which has all the raw materials for a new human life. This is called **fertilization**. It happens in the oviduct.

The fertilized egg begins its journey to the womb. It starts growing by dividing – 2 cells, then 4, 8, 16, 32, and so on. After about five days, it reaches the womb as a tiny ball of many cells. The tiny ball attaches itself to the rich lining of the womb. This is called **implantation**, which comes from the verb 'to implant'.

When human life begins

Some people believe human life begins at fertilization. Others believe it begins at implantation. Still others believe it does not begin until birth – or until about 28 weeks after fertilization when the baby could be **viable** (able to live outside the womb). The normal date of birth is counted as 280 days or 40 weeks from the *first* day of the woman's last period. All couples, whether using family planning or trying for a baby, should keep a record of the woman's monthly cycle.

How family planning works

Study the diagram on p. 122 carefully. Try to keep clear in your mind the passage of the sperms to the oviduct and then work out the passage of the fertilized egg to the womb. Family planning works by stopping the sperms and egg meeting – there is *no* fertilization. Or it works by stopping the fertilized egg from becoming implanted in the womb – there is *no* implantation.

Moral attitudes to family planning

In certain cultures or religions, family planning is considered morally wrong. In other cultures, only the methods which stop fertilization are allowed. Each person's opinion has to be respected. For example, when do *you* think human life begins? Perhaps it would be helpful to have a full discussion on this now.

Mixed feelings about family planning

As yet, there is no one perfect method of family planning – apart from abstinence. All the methods require some kind of discipline and self-control. For example, if the woman uses the pill, she must remember to take it; if the man uses the sheath, he must remember to buy supplies. Also, some methods carry the risk of unpleasant side effects.

Some couples are very keen to control their fertility. They make sure they have proper protection. Others, often young couples, do not want a baby but dislike the bother and fuss. Each month they go through endless worry, waiting for the woman's period to start. This can damage their love – in extreme cases, it can damage their lives (p. 138).

Infertility

This means being unable to start a baby. About one in ten couples are infertile. The man may not produce enough fertile sperm, or his sperm tubes may be blocked. The woman may not produce fertile eggs, or her oviducts may be blocked. There are other reasons for infertility. In many cases the couple can be treated at a fertility clinic. New techniques in surgery make it possible for sperms and egg to meet in a glass tube outside the woman's body. The ball of cells can then be implanted in her womb. This operation is not suitable for all infertile couples.

Points for discussion
1   Some people think that any method of family planning interferes with nature and is morally wrong.
2   Some people think that a couple who have more than two children (replacing themselves) are greedy and selfish as the world is already over-populated and other people are starving to death.

Questions

1   **Copy the diagram into your book and label it.**
2   **In your own words, describe what happens at fertilization.**
3   **What are the two main ways in which family planning works?**
4   **What is infertility? Write a few sentences about it.**

Family planning methods (1)

1 Natural methods

'Natural' here means not using anything which is 'artificial'. The couple control their fertility by careful timing with their love-making and a great deal of self-discipline. Natural methods usually work better in older couples who are *very* keen not to start a baby, and who keep careful records.

Male withdrawal

This is sometimes called 'being careful'. The man withdraws his penis before emission so there is no semen inside the woman. Withdrawal is the oldest and most widely used method throughout the world. Older couples may prefer it as it is a simple matter between them, and there are no side effects.

For young couples, however, withdrawal often fails. It is quite difficult for a young man to have enough control to be completely 'careful'. Even one drop of semen leaked will contain millions of sperms. Also, there can be emotional side effects from this method. One or both partners may be tense and unhappy in case it fails.

The calendar or rhythm method

This used to be called the 'safe period'. It is based on the woman's monthly cycle. Love-making only happens during her *infertile* time. This is when there is no egg in the oviduct, so she needs to learn the signs when there *is* an egg present. Her body temperature rises slightly and there are changes in her vaginal juices. At the clinic, she will be taught how to notice these changes, and her fertile/infertile calendar will be worked out.

Some older couples prefer this method as it is based on the woman's natural body rhythms. But it can be difficult to work out her calendar and she must have very regular monthly periods. Young couples can also use this method – its success will depend upon how keen they are not to start a baby.

2 Barrier methods

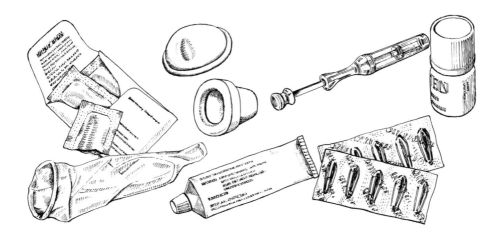

These are ways of stopping the sperms from getting to the egg by using artificial barriers. They have no side effects, and only require a little self-control. The man must stop love-making to put on the condom or the woman must put in her cap before love-making starts. Spermicides (chemicals which kill sperms) are also a barrier method.

The condom (man)

The condom is also called the sheath, French letter, protective, and so on. It is made of thin rubber and in one size, which can stretch. There is a rim at one end and a teat to trap the semen at the other. It can only be put on after the man has an erection. After love-making, the man must remove himself carefully, holding the rim of the condom close against his body so no semen escapes. This is *very* important.

The condom is a popular method of family planning as it is a private matter between the couple. It fails if it breaks or if it is not removed carefully enough. To be safe, it is better if the woman puts spermicide inside her vagina. There are short condoms which only cover the glans. They may slip off, or fit too tightly. They are not safe.

The cap (woman)

This is a rubber barrier which covers the entrance to the cervix. It comes in different sizes and shapes – the diaphragm is the cap most widely used. The woman must be measured for size, and shown how to put it in place. She must also cover it with spermicide cream in case any sperms manage to get around the rim. After childbirth, her size must be checked again as it is likely she will need a slightly larger size.

The cap is a popular method of family planning for the woman who does not want to take pills. It must be put in place before love-making, and left there for at least six hours after. Then it is removed, washed in warm soapy water, and gently dried. It is examined for holes through which the sperms could swim, and put away until next time.

Spermicides (woman)

These include creams, aerosol foams, jellies, and suppositories (tablets which melt in the vagina). They are *not* safe on their own – but they are better than nothing at all. The most recent one is a sponge soaked in spermicide. This is moistened and put high up in the vagina before love-making. It is safer than the others as the sponge opens out to block the entrance to the cervix. But to be really safe, the man should use a condom or the woman a cap at the same time.

Questions

1 **Explain why the withdrawal method is not very safe for young couples.**
2 **In your own words, explain what is meant by the calendar or rhythm method and say why the woman must go to the clinic.**
3 **Name two precautions the couple must take when using the condom.**
4 **Why must a spermicide cream always be used with the cap?**

Family planning methods (2)

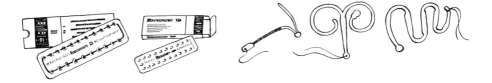

3 The combined pill (woman)

These tablets are based on the two female sex hormones, oestrogen and progesterone. They work by stopping the normal hormone changes of the monthly cycle so that an egg is not developed or released from the ovary. The combined pill must be taken daily for three weeks, then stopped for one week. This stopping causes a period, which is lighter than normal. The combined pill is the most effective method of family planning. It is very powerful and the woman must go for regular check-ups on her health.

The mini-pill (woman)

The combined pill is not suitable for young girls, especially if their periods have not settled down. The mini-pill is based on only one female sex hormone, progesterone. It works in a different way from the combined pill. An egg is released from the ovary so the periods are natural. The mini-pill must be taken every day at the same time throughout the monthly cycle.

The problems

The combined pill carries a slight risk of thrombosis (p. 38) – a greater tendency to form blood clots in the arteries and veins. Other side effects may include raised blood pressure (p. 94), headaches, thrush (p.141), and feeling slightly dizzy or sick. Women who are over 35, who smoke, or who are overweight should not take the combined pill.

    The mini-pill is not as effective as the combined pill, but the side effects are fewer. Blood clotting is not affected. The monthly bleeding pattern tends to be erratic. Women over 35 can take the mini-pill. However, there is a risk of cancer of the uterus and breast cancer (p. 153) from both kinds of pills, especially in young women, or those taking the pill for more than a few years.

    Some women do not have any side effects, whichever pill they take. But if a woman does have side effects and they do not wear off, it is wiser to try another method of family planning. The problems of side effects have to be weighed against how keen the couple are to control their fertility.

4 The IUD (woman)

IUD stands for **intra-uterine device**. This means a coil, loop, or copper-7 which is eased through the cervix and put into the womb. The IUD works by stopping the tiny ball of cells becoming implanted in the womb. IUDs come in different sizes and a coloured string is left hanging into the top of the vagina. Blue is for the smallest, then black, yellow, white, according to the woman's size and whether she has already had babies.

Fitting the IUD

This must be done by a trained person, though not always a doctor. The best time to be fitted is during or just after a period, but it can be done at any time. Some IUDs stay in place and are only removed when the couple want to start their family. Others must be taken out and replaced after a certain time. The woman is taught how to feel the coloured string to make sure the IUD is still in place. In a few women the IUD is pushed out, usually quite soon after the fitting.

The problems

There will be a little bleeding, there may be a few cramps, and the next periods are likely to be rather heavy. But these things settle down after the first few months. If they do not, then the IUD is removed and another method may be tried. There is also a slight risk of infection (pelvic inflammatory disease, p. 140) as germs may travel up the string into the womb. But in terms of not starting a baby, the IUD is the next safest method after the pill.

5 Sterilization (man or woman)

The sperm tubes of the man or the oviducts of the woman are cut and tied back. Sterilization is only for older couples who already have a family.

Safety factors

Charts showing how safe the different methods are have now been stopped. They could not be worked out accurately. When family planning fails, for whatever reason, it is natural to blame the method rather than the way the couple used it. However, the pill is very safe indeed – if it is always taken. The IUD is almost as safe, though not quite. The barrier methods give good protection if a spermicide is used with the condom or the cap. The condom also gives some – though not much – protection against sexual disease (pp. 140–1). The natural methods are the least safe of all. They require self-discipline and a very keen desire to control fertility if they are to work.

Points to consider
1   The safest methods of family planning in terms of not starting a baby carry the greatest risks of side effects.
2   Though a couple may choose their method of family planning together, the woman takes the greater risk if it fails, or if it has side effects.

Questions

1   **Name three groups of women for whom the combined pill is not advised.**
2   **Using the page references given in the text, try to work out why women who smoke or who are overweight may have a greater tendency to develop thrombosis.**
3   **Name the problems which may happen when using an IUD.**
4   **Of all the methods of family planning, which do you think might be the most popular? Perhaps it would be helpful to have a discussion on this.**

About family planning failure

Taking risks

Young couples with mixed feelings about family planning sometimes take risks. They make love without proper protection. They need to remember that with each emission of semen about 200,000,000 sperms go chasing after the egg! *This will happen from puberty onwards.* The old wives' tales about not starting a baby the first time, or the girl coughing, standing up, or passing water immediately afterwards, *do not work.*

'What will be, will be'

The first signs of pregnancy include missed periods, tingling or swelling of the breasts, and early morning sickness. Couples with mixed feelings about family planning may be secretly delighted when they notice these signs. 'It was meant to be,' they think, and settle down happily to married life and parenthood.

The 'morning after' pill

But some couples are extremely anxious not to start a baby. If, for example, the condom bursts, the woman can go to the clinic as soon as possible after love making. The 'morning after' pills are especially high doses of one or both of the female sex hormones. They usually have unpleasant side effects. They are used for emergency situations and are *not* another method of family planning. In some women, for example those who have had children, an IUD may be inserted to prevent implantation of the egg.

Abortion

This is also called termination of pregnancy. A pregnancy can be terminated (stopped) by medical means. The reasons include rape (sexual intercourse by force); cases where tests show the unborn baby is damaged; and where it is thought that the woman's mental or physical health, and/or the welfare of her family, will suffer is she has to continue an unplanned pregnancy.

How abortions are done

1 When a woman has missed her period for 14 days or less, a small tube can be passed through the cervix into the womb. The contents are syringed out under vacuum pressure. This is called **menstrual regulation**.
2 From 14 days up to 12 weeks, the woman needs an anaesthetic (powerful pain killer). The cervix has to be opened before the contents of the womb can be removed.
3 After 12 weeks, fluids which start labour (birth) are dripped into the woman's arm through a needle. After the 'birth', the womb may have to be scraped out to make sure all the contents have come away.

Attitudes to abortion

Though laws have been passed to allow termination of pregnancy, many people are still horrified at the thought of abortion. The couple themselves may be in deep despair, and suffer great anguish over what they should do. It is as well to remember in any discussion about abortion that no one really *likes* it. Abortion is usually the last desperate step in what has often been a whole series of muddles and mistakes.

Counselling

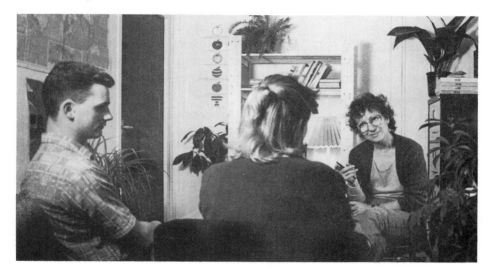

Before any decision can be made, the couple will be counselled – given advice and offered support. It is important the woman's true feelings are known. She may secretly want the baby but be afraid her partner does not. She may so dislike the idea of abortion, she prefers to have the baby and then give it for adoption. These things must be worked out, if possible, first.

Women who really want an abortion feel tremendous relief afterwards. Those who were unhappy about it are likely to feel quite 'bad' for some time after. Unfortunately, the decision has to be made in rather a hurry. Late abortions – after 12 weeks – are rarely advised.

Points to discuss
1 Some people think that doctors who perform abortions and the women who have them are guilty of murder of the unborn child.
2 Some people think that termination of pregnancy is a kind and caring way of helping people who are in great distress.

Questions

1 **What do the first signs of pregnancy include?**
2 **In your own words, write about the 'morning after' pill.**
3 **Do you think it important teenagers should know about abortion? Give as many reasons as you can for your answer.**

Sexually transmitted diseases (STDs)

STDs (venereal diseases) are the harsher side of love. In the under-nineteen-year olds, they have risen steadily in recent years.

1 **Gonorrhoea**
Men: Burning pain when passing water; smelly discharge from penis.
Women: Heavy discharge, some pain; but seventy per cent have no symptoms.
If the disease is not treated, bacteria breed in the sperm tubes and oviducts. These get blocked and the person becomes sterile. Gonorrhoea is rising steadily amongst young people.

2 **Non-specific urethritis (NSU)**
Men only: The same symptoms as gonorrhoea, but it is not understood what causes it. If untreated, NSU can lead to infections of the eyes, skin, and mouth, and to painful diseases of the joints. NSU is also on the increase among young men.

3 **Pelvic inflammatory disease (PID)**
Women only: Acute or burning pain caused by infection of the oviducts. It is caused by bacteria which attack the oviducts, making them swollen and very sore. If untreated, PID blocks the oviducts and the woman becomes sterile. PID is also on the increase among young women.

4 **Herpes**
These look rather like 'cold sores' on or inside the sex organs. Herpes are caused by virus germs and can be very difficult to treat. The sores vanish but then re-appear at regular intervals. It is thought they cause other damage, especially in women. Herpes is increasing at an alarming rate among young people.

5 **Syphilis**
Men: Painless sore on sex organs which vanishes after a few weeks.
Women: Painless sore on or inside the sex organs which also vanishes. If untreated, the bacteria enter the blood stream and cause hidden damage. Later in life this leads to insanity, blindness, paralysis, and eventually death. Syphilis is now on the decrease.

6 **Trichomonas vaginalis**
Women only: yellow smelly discharge; pain, itchiness, sore sex organs. If untreated, the condition becomes chronic (permanent low infection).

7 **Warts**
These look like tiny cauliflowers on the sex organs, and are caused by virus germs. Any infection of the sex organs must be treated immediately to stop other germs getting in (secondary infection).

8 **Scabies**
Tiny parasites which burrow under the skin and lay eggs. They breed quickly in warm damp areas of the body. There is a risk of secondary infection. (See p. 27.)

9 **Lice**
Tiny parasites which stick on to pubic hair. Very itchy. (See p. 26.)

10 **Candidiosis (thrush)**
Men: Penis red and sore at tip. Men rarely have it.
Women: Thick discharge, sore and itchy vagina.
Thrush is not always caught sexually. It is a fungus infection which can be caused by other things, e.g. certain medicines. If untreated, the condition becomes chronic.

Facts about STDs

1 STDs are passed directly from one person to another. They are not caught from toilet seats or towels – the germs die when not on the human body.
2 Gonorrhoea, herpes, and syphilis can all damage the baby, either before or during birth.
3 STDs are treated at special clinics attached to most hospitals. Many people prefer not to go to their family doctor, though treatment is private in both places.
4 People who start their sex life early and who have many changes of partners are at much greater risk of catching an STD.
5 Most STDs can be cured it they are treated as soon as the symptoms are noticed. The longer the person waits, the more difficult the treatment.
6 A person can be a 'carrier' without having any symptoms. Love-making must stop immediately if the partner notices something wrong. *Both* people should go to the special clinic for a check-up. This is very important to stop any chance of re-infection.
7 Pain on passing water, or an unpleasant discharge, do not necessarily mean the person has an STD. But both these symptoms show something is going wrong which needs to be put right.
8 For any worry, a visit to the special clinic is helpful. This is especially so for women if they fear there is a chance of disease inside the vagina, which they cannot see. If there is no cause for alarm, the visit is not wasted. Peace of mind about personal health is very important indeed.

A quote to consider
'The most important fact about the sexually transmitted diseases is that they are not contracted (caught) by people *who have only one sexual partner.'*
(*Dr R.D. Catterall*, IPPF Medical Publications)

Questions

1 **What are the symptoms of gonorrhoea?**
2 **What happens if (a) NSU and (b) PID are not treated?**
3 **Name the two skin infections caused by tiny parasites.**
4 **Can STDs be caught from toilet seats? Give a reason for your answer.**
5 **Where do people go for treatment of an STD?**

Further work on Chapter 4

1 Conflicts with adults are fairly usual in the teens. Write an essay, discussing some of the reasons for this.

2 Describe (a) a *mild* conflict you had with adults in which you won and (b) one in which you lost. Explain the reasons for the different results.

3 A few teenage groups cut out adult company completely. In what ways might this be harmful if it happens over a long period of time?

4 What is meant by 'deviant' behaviour? Why do adults sometimes worry about teenagers 'getting in with the wrong group'?

5 It is difficult to hold out against peer group pressure in the teens. Do you agree with this statement, or not? Give reasons for your answer.

6 Write about the importance of genital hygiene in the teens.

7 Discuss the differences in a man's and a woman's fertile life.

8 Some teenagers are fully fertile by the mid-teens. Do you think this means they are ready for the responsibilities of young adult life? (p. 12).

9 'Coping with pressures' (p. 127) is about the sexual double standard. For example: girls are still called unpleasant names if they are promiscuous, whereas boys are not. Have a discussion on this.

10 What is the total number of schoolgirls who are pregnant each year by the age of 16?

11 One in three marriages break down (a) when people marry under 20, and (b) when there is a baby already on the way. Write an essay, discussing the reasons why you think these marriages have less chance of being successful.

12 Find out where the local Marriage Guidance office is. If possible, visit them and write an account of their work.

13 What do you consider are the most important qualities in (a) a future husband, and (b) a future wife? Why?

14 If possible, visit a register office. Copy out the exact vows the couple make to each other.

15 Visit your local family planning clinic, or write with a stamped addressed envelope for their leaflets. Study the contents and do a full project on the different methods.

16 A couple are too shy to go to a family planning clinic. What methods of birth control could they use by shopping at the chemist's?

17 Find out under what conditions a woman may have an abortion. Do you agree, or disagree, with those conditions? Have a discussion on this.

18 From what you have learned about sexually-transmitted diseases, why is faithfulness between couples so important in terms of health?

Chapter 5

About community health

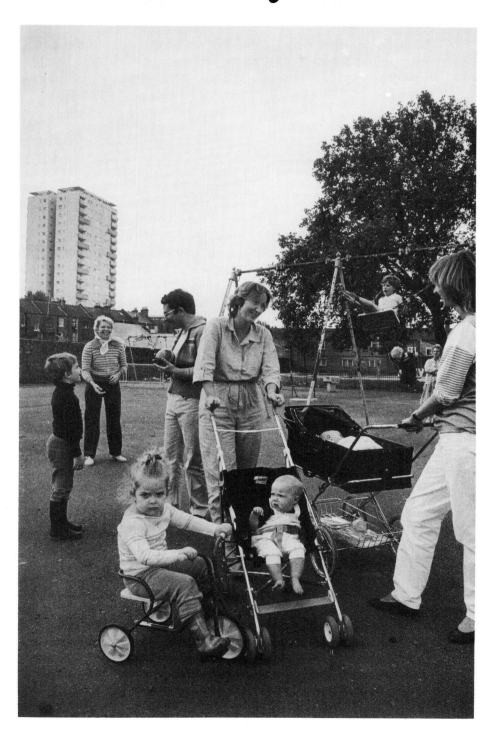

Genes and inherited illness

About genes

Genes pass down family likeness – the things you inherit from your parents.
They are like tiny beads on chains inside the nucleus of cells. Before
fertilization, the genes are shuffled around inside each sperm and each egg.
They 'set' in a definite pattern the moment the sperm fertilizes the egg.

Why you are 'unique'

You inherit equal amounts of genes from each parent. But you only get half
your mother's and half your father's – which is why you are different from them
both. Also, because of the shuffling around before fertilization, you get different
genes 'set' in a different pattern – this is why you are different from your sisters
and brothers.

The things you inherit

You inherit such things as body shape, blood group, general intelligence, and
the risks of certain illnesses. Not all the things you inherit are known. This is
because some genes are **dominant** – they mask or hide the effects of the
others. But you will be carrying the others. They are called **recessive** genes. If
you marry a person who has the same recessive genes, then the hidden effects
have a chance to show through in your baby.

Dominant	*Recessive*
short height	tall height
kinky hair	curly hair
curly hair	straight hair
dark skin	light skin
dark eyes	light eyes
large nose	small nose

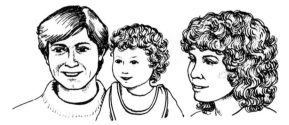

Inherited illness

If you fall in love with someone who has an inherited illness in the family, or if
you yourself are in that position – what should you do? Lovers can be wildly
romantic, and decide to ignore such dreadful things. In olden days, they hid
away handicapped babies and told fearful tales of 'bad' blood. Young couples
with special worries – for example, a handicapped person in either family –
should go to a Genetic Counselling Clinic long before a baby is started.

Genetic counselling

A dominant gene for an inherited illness carries the risk of one in two children
being affected. Two recessive genes carry the risk of one in four children
having the illness. But genes are very complicated things to work out. Only
highly skilled experts can estimate the risks. And there is always the chance
the couple will find out the illness is not inherited at all.

But if it is, the couple need to understand the problems they face. Some parents are wonderful at looking after handicapped babies. Others are not. The staff at the clinic explain what the illness is like, whether it can be treated or cured, and what kinds of special care the baby will need. Once the couple have this information, they can decide whether to start a family, or not.

Testing for handicap

Amniocentesis is the name of a test which can be done after 16 weeks of pregnancy. A small amount of the 'waters' the baby lies in is taken from the mother's womb through a needle. This is tested and, if handicap is found, the couple are offered a termination of pregnancy. The couple can then decide if they want to continue the pregnancy, or not. The test itself carries a very slight risk that early labour might start. Can you see why it is better to go to a Genetic Counselling Clinic *before* starting a baby if there are special reasons for worry?

Down's syndrome

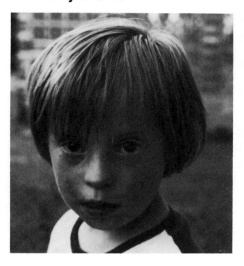

This is the name for what used to be called a mongol baby. Down's syndrome is *not* an inherited condition. A Down's baby has small eyes which slant upwards, a short flat nose, and a thick tongue which tends to stick out. The baby is mentally handicapped (p. 156) but can learn slowly. Some will always need special care. The risk of having a Down's syndrome baby increases with the age of the mother.

Mother's age	The risk	Mother's age	The risk
20–24	1 in 2,000	35–39	1 in 300
25–29	1 in 1,500	40–44	1 in 100
30–34	1 in 1,000	45+	1 in 50

Questions

1 **Are you a 'chip off the old block'? Describe the things you think you may have inherited from (a) your mother and (b) your father.**
2 **Explain what is meant by 'dominant' and 'recessive' genes. Give examples of each.**
3 **What advice would you give to a couple with special worries about handicap?**
4 **Do you think you could look after a handicapped baby? Give reasons for your answer.**

Starting a family

There is no such time as the 'best' time to start a family. People are different. Some couples long for a baby soon after marriage. Other couples want to wait until they have a comfortable home. And still others prefer not to have children at all. During courtship, the decisions about having babies should be discussed by the couple. These decisions include:

(a) *if* the couple want children;
(b) *when* the couple would like to have children;
(c) *how many* children the couple would like to have.

Very young parents

Babies need a great deal of care and personal attention. A few very young parents do not understand how changed their lives will be once the baby arrives. They may feel unhappy about losing their youth and their freedom. They may feel trapped if they have to stay at home night after night. There is a risk they may turn their unhappy feelings onto the baby.

Many teenage couples make marvellous parents. But the tragic cases of 'baby-battering' are often the result of parents not understanding how a baby will change their lives.

Much older parents

Having a baby late in life also carries certain risks. The older the mother, the greater the chance of Down's Syndrome (p. 145), mental handicap (p. 156), poor physical development, and early labour. Older fathers too are linked with certain kinds of poor development while the baby is in the womb.

But the longing to have a baby can be very powerful. Many older parents are prepared to take these risks because they want a baby so much. Often, they are rewarded with a perfectly healthy baby.

Unhappy couples

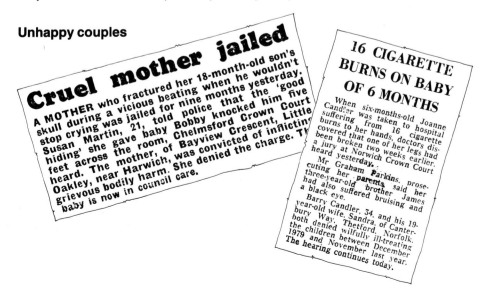

Cruel mother jailed

A MOTHER who fractured her 18-month-old son's skull during a vicious beating when he wouldn't stop crying was jailed for nine months yesterday.

Susan Martin, 21, told police that the 'good hiding' she gave baby Bobby knocked him five feet across the room, Chelmsford Crown Court heard. The mother, of Bayview Crescent, Little Oakley, near Harwich, was convicted of inflicting grievous bodily harm. She denied the charge. The baby is now in council care.

16 CIGARETTE BURNS ON BABY OF 6 MONTHS

When six-months-old Joanne Candler was taken to hospital suffering from 16 cigarette burns to her hands, doctors discovered that one of her legs had been broken two weeks earlier, a jury at Norwich Crown Court heard yesterday.

Mr Graham Parkins, prosecuting her parents, said her three-year-old brother James had also suffered bruising and a black eye.

Barry Candler, 34, and his 19-year-old wife, Sandra, of Canterbury Way, Thetford, Norfolk, both denied wilfully ill-treating the children between December 1979 and November last year. The hearing continues today.

Some couples decide to have a baby to 'patch up the marriage'. But babies are very hard work – there are bound to be some sleepless nights during the first months. Unhappy parents are likely to have very tense feelings about each other. Sleepless nights added to the extra work may make them feel even more tense and unhappy.

There are rare cases where a baby has drawn the parents closer together. But more often, the baby suffers from neglect, or lack of love, or cruel words and harsh blows. This is called **child abuse**.

Babies close together

Mothers and babies are likely to have safer pregnancies if there is a gap of two years between the birth of each child. Having babies closer together than this is called **close parity**. But some parents want large families and have a new baby each year, and each baby is born more healthy than the last. Knowing about the very slight risk of close parity is general advice to parents who want to know whether to have their babies close together or space them out.

Starting a family

This is a very exciting time. The couple do not have to bother with family planning. Their love-making may be more deep and profound because they are hoping to create a new life. But if the woman has been using the pill, it may take a little while for her hormones to settle down again. And not all babies choose to be conceived at the exact moment that their parents wish!

Couples need not be upset if there are no immediate signs of pregnancy (p. 138). They can enjoy going on trying for a baby for six months without worrying. In fact, some doctors think couples can try for much longer without fears of being infertile (p. 133).

For discussion:
Basil and Bertha are madly in love. He comes from a large family and wants one of his own. Bertha dislikes babies. She wants to do well in her career. They do not discuss this difference openly. They marry, each secretly hoping they can change the other's mind.

Do you think they are likely to have a successful marriage? What are the choices they can make now?

Questions

1 **During courtship, what are the three decisions about having babies couples should discuss? Explain why you think these decisions are important *before* marriage.**
2 **Name some of the reasons why a few very young parents may turn against their babies.**
3 **What are the health risks much older parents face when they start a baby?**
4 **What is meant by 'close parity'? As it is only a very slight risk, why is it mentioned here?**

Antenatal care

'Ante' means before and 'natal' means birth. It is important that a woman goes for antenatal care as soon as she thinks she is pregnant (p. 138). Having a baby does not mean being ill. But there are certain things which can harm the new human life. When a baby is planned, the woman can avoid these risks.

Things which can harm an unborn baby

1 **Drugs** Certain drugs will damage the baby's development. No medicines of any kind should be taken unless they are prescribed by a doctor.
2 **Smoking and drinking** As these are drugs, they can damage the baby. Heavy smokers or drinkers should try to stop before becoming pregnant.
3 **X-rays** If a woman thinks she is pregnant and needs an X-ray, she must tell the hospital staff. A protective shield will be used.
4 **Rubella (German measles)** This is a mild disease in adults but causes terrible damage in an unborn baby. Girls of 11 to 13 are now vaccinated against rubella to prevent this happening.
5 **STDs** Sexual diseases can harm the baby either before or during birth. If a mother thinks she may have an infection, she should ask for tests to be carried out. She can then be treated, and no harm will be done.
6 **Life crisis** This is any big change which causes stress – moving house, losing a job, getting divorced, a death in the family. Mothers who are under stress from life crises may have less well-developed babies.
7 A young single girl, with no money and no home, living on hand-outs from friends and moving from 'squat' to 'squat', is less likely to have a healthy baby and to be healthy herself.
8 A woman whose husband drinks and is violent, and who cares for her three other children by scrubbing office floors, is less likely to have a healthy baby and to be healthy herself.

At the antenatal clinic

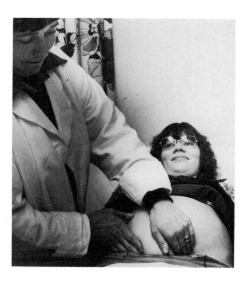

1 The mother's blood and urine are tested to see if all is well.
2 Her blood pressure is regularly checked to make sure it stays low.
3 Her weight increase is watched – she must not put on too much or too little.
4 Her medical 'history' and her husband's will be written down.
5 Later on, the baby's heart beat is listened to for a good steady beat.
6 Advice on diet, exercise, rest, and anything which might be worrying the mother will be given.
7 Both she and her husband can attend classes to learn about the birth and caring for the new baby.

Home or hospital?

First babies are usually born in the **maternity ward** of a hospital. And mothers who are over 35, or who have a 'history' of health problems, have their babies in maternity wards too. Early in pregnancy, the mother's bed is booked. She is given a **certificate of expected confinement** at 26 weeks. This gives the date when the baby is expected. She is also given an exemption for payment card for free dental treatment, free milk and vitamins, and free medicines – if they are needed.

Some mothers want their second babies to be born at home. This is called a **home confinement**. The mother is looked after by a **midwife**. Home confinements carry a slight risk in case something goes wrong and the mother has to be rushed to hospital. A few people who do not like hospitals and prefer the comfort of being in familiar surroundings are willing to take this risk. But home confinements are still very rare – especially in communities a long way from a central hospital.

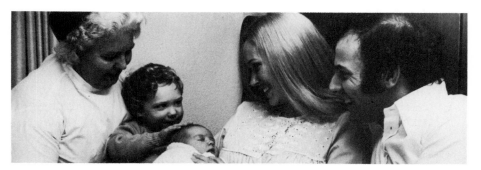

People the mother may meet

1   The **family doctor** is usually the first person the mother sees. She will be given an internal examination and her pregnancy will be confirmed.
2   Most **midwives** are fully trained nurses with extra training in pregnancy and childbirth. The midwife looks after the mother before, during, and for a few days after the birth.
3   The **health visitor** is a fully trained nurse with extra training in child care and general family health. She visits the family regularly after the birth.
4   The **social worker** has special training in the welfare of the family and the community. Families in difficulty may need practical help such as food, clothing, or a roof over their heads.
5   The **paediatrician** is a doctor who specializes in children's health. If there is something wrong with the new baby, the paediatrician will help.

Questions

1   **Write a list of the stresses you think a single mother who is 16 is likely to be under. In what ways may these stresses affect her baby?**
2   **Which do you think better, a home or hospital confinement? Try to answer from as many points of view as you can.**
3   **Copy out the list of people the mother may meet. Learn the work of each person who helps with the new family.**

About healthy children

Averages

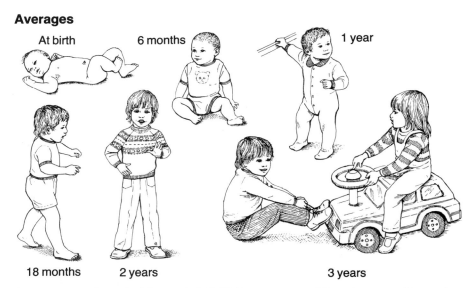

At birth   6 months   1 year

18 months   2 years   3 years

Average new-born babies weigh 3.5 kilograms, are 50 cm long, and have large heads for their body size. By six months, they are twice their birth weight and the body is getting larger in proportion to the head. At one year, they should have trebled their birth weight and their bodies are longer and stronger.

Average toddlers will walk without support before the age of 18 months. By two years they can say 50 words but understand many more. By the third birthday, they need the company of other children. At about five, they are ready to begin learning: reading, writing, and sums.

Milestones

These stages in a child's development are called **milestones**. Milestones are averages – there is no such person as an average child. The rate at which babies develop will depend upon the genes they inherit. It will also depend upon the environment – whether there is love, good care, and things to interest the growing mind.

Regular check-ups

Milestones of development are checked at Mother and Baby Clinics or Child Health Centres. Parents need to remember milestones are only guidelines. They are *not* rules. The health visitor weighs the baby, checks for general development, and watches for signs of anything going wrong. She notes the baby's mental development too. Does he smile at his mother? Is he looking bright and alert?

The importance of regular check-ups

A baby with hearing problems cannot listen to words and so will be very backward at learning to talk. A baby with partial sight cannot reach for a toy and so will be very backward at learning to read and write. Both these babies could have been helped if they were taken to the clinic for regular check-ups. Anything which is going wrong needs to be found out as early as possible. Things which are not put right nearly always cause new – and more difficult – problems later on.

Immunization

Babies have little natural protection against germs. Terrible diseases such as smallpox and diphtheria used to kill thousands of babies each year. Nowadays, attacks of diphtheria are very rare and smallpox has been wiped out completely. This is because of world-wide immunization, which makes babies immune (safe) from attack.

Very weak or dead germs are given to the baby. During immunization the baby's body builds up defences against the disease. As the child gets older, he is given booster (extra) shots. These make sure his body defences stay immune from the disease.

Average times for immunization

1. The 'triple' immunization against diphtheria, whooping cough, and tetanus is given at about three, five and nine months of age. The booster shot is given at the age of 4½–5½.
2. The polio immunization is given at the same time, but not by injection. It is given as drops direct to babies, and drops on a lump of sugar to older children.
3. A booster dose of tetanus and polio vaccine is offered to school-leavers.
4. The vaccine against measles is given during the child's second year.
5. The rubella (German measles) vaccine is offered to girls between 11 and 13. This is before puberty. Turn to page 148 to check why.
6. The BCG vaccine against tuberculosis is given between 10 and 15 but only after a skin test to find out if it is needed.

The school health service

This gives regular medical check-ups to children in school. Parents are invited to attend as well. The child's general progress is tested to make sure he or she is developing well. There are dental inspections, visits by school nurses, school clinics, and health education officers. The child guidance clinic will look after the child's mental health.

Free education and the school welfare services continue to look after the needs of growing children. There are many other ways in which society looks after the health, happiness, and proper development of babies and children.

Questions

1. **What is meant by 'milestones'? Give two examples.**
2. **In your own words, explain the importance of regular check-ups.**
3. **Copy out the average times for immunization.**
4. **Write a short essay about some of the ways in which society looks after the health, happiness, and proper development of babies and children.**

About healthy adults

Preventive health work

Many diseases can be treated and cured if they are discovered early. Testing blood pressure may show the beginnings of a heart problem. X-rays show the early stages of lung cancer or tuberculosis – before the person feels ill. Lorries fitted with X-ray machines are called **mobile units**. They visit factories, offices, and schools to check on the health of people's lungs.

A complete check-up

Before you start work, you may need a complete medical check-up. Careers which require this include the police, the armed forces, the medical profession, and many other jobs which involve working with people. If you want a really tough career – working on an oil rig or down the mines – you will need to prove you are physically fit. Also, when you take out a life insurance policy, the company may ask you to have a complete medical check-up.

Your general appearance

The doctor is likely to measure your height and weight first. During this time, notice is taken of your general appearance. Have you good posture, clear eyes, a healthy skin? Are you bright and alert? Is your speech clear and distinct? Most people do not enjoy being physically examined. The doctor takes into account the fact you may be feeling slightly nervous – even though there is nothing wrong with you.

1   Your breathing and heart-beats are listened to through a **stethoscope**. Say '99'. There will be wheezes if you smoke. Your heart should give clear, sharp, distinct beats.

2   Your lung expansion may be measured and your chest wall thumped. Normal lungs give a different sound from damaged ones.

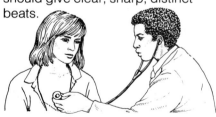

3   Your blood pressure is measured and your pulse rate is taken.

4   Your reflexes, such as the knee jerk, will be tested. Then your spine and limbs will be examined for any problems in the blood vessels, bones, and joints.

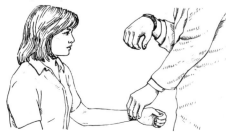

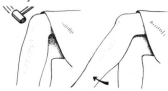

5   This person is having her ear-drums checked.

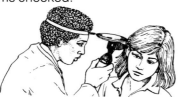

6   Say 'Aaah!' Tongue, tonsils, and throat are examined.

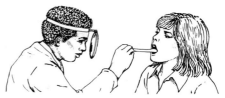

7   An **ophthalmoscope** is used to look inside your eyes at the back lining. The light is shone to see if your pupils get smaller.

8   Your neck and throat are felt for swollen glands. The glands in your armpits and groin may also be felt.

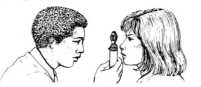

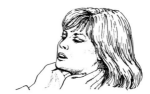

9   Your abdomen is examined. The doctor's hands feel for lumps, or for an enlarged liver, kidney, or spleen.

10   The reproductive organs and back passage are also examined.

11   You stand up and cough to make sure there is no hernia (rupture) of the abdomen wall.

12   You may be sent for a chest X-ray.

13   You may give blood and urine samples. A great deal about your state of health can be learned from tests done on them.

For women

1   Breasts are examined for lumps. The woman may be offered an **infra-red scan**. Areas where there is cancer have a slightly higher temperature than the rest of the body. An infra-red scan 'photographs' the breasts in colour.

2   She may be given a **cervical smear**. This means the cervix is lightly scraped (it does not hurt) and the cells examined under a microscope. Any unhealthy cells will be noticed (p. 96). Women over the age of 35 are advised to have a cervical smear every two years. Younger women can have them done less frequently. The family doctor or the staff at the family planning clinic will give advice on this.

3   Women, whatever their age, who have been using the pill, are advised to have regular checks against both breast cancer and cancer of the cervix.

Questions

1   **Explain how mobile X-ray units keep a check on the community's health.**

2   **Name two reasons why you may need a complete medical check-up.**

3   **Some life insurance policies cost more if you smoke. Have a discussion on whether this is fair, or not.**

4   **Re-read the first paragraph and turn to page 96. Write a few lines, explaining what a cervical smear is and why it is so important women have one done regularly.**

About healthy ageing

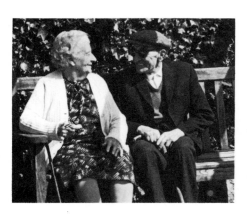

When are people old?

Men usually retire from work at 65 and women at 60. This is the official time when you are considered old. But life expectancy is rising. Now it is 70 for men and 77 for women. By the year 2050, it is expected to reach the mid 80s. A quarter of your life could be spent in healthy active retirement. Do you think, perhaps, we should not regard people as old until they reach their three score years and ten?

Attitudes to the elderly

At whatever age, human life is precious. We all have the right to our dignity and self-respect. But old people are often treated as if they had no feelings at all. They are called 'Gran' and 'Grandad' by strangers. They still have personal names. They are still Mrs and Mr Smith; Mary and Bob. They may be thought of as useless, and a great expense to the state. But they have worked hard and earned their pensions. Many are very active and extremely useful members of the community.

Where the elderly live

70% of people over 65 live with their families.
24% manage to stay in their own homes.
  3% live in residential homes for the elderly.
  3% stay in hospital. They need special full-time care.

There is a general idea that families do not care for their elderly. These figures show this is not true. Grown-up children take on the responsibility of looking after their ageing parents. Family ties of love and duty are very strong indeed.

The ageing process

Human bodies are rather like machines. They suffer from general wear and tear over the years. This does not mean, however, that to be old is to be ill. Many elderly people are fit, active, and alert until their last days. They adjust to the normal health problems of growing old.

1 **Sight** From about the age of 40, eyesight is less good. Spectacles may be needed for reading and close work. Later on, certain diseases can damage the sight. Regular check-ups at the optician's are important.
2 **Hearing and balance** Over the years, these become less good. One in eight people between the ages of 65 and 75 have hearing problems. This rises to one in four at 75+. Hearing aids can be used, and hurried movements slowed down.

3 **Mobility** Bones can become thin and brittle. They break easily after a fall. Arthritis in the leg or hip can stiffen up the joints. Hands which once were graceful may become gnarled and painful. Feet which marched into battle may be tender and sore.

Help for the elderly

1 **Sight** In the day-time, curtains should be drawn right back to let in natural light. In the evenings, bright artificial lights are needed instead of dim lamps. A magnifying glass can be left by the telephone. An extra pair of spectacles is useful in case the first pair breaks.
2 **Hearing** During conversation, cut out all background noise. A slightly deaf person cannot hear if the radio or television is left on. Always talk clearly and directly (face to face) with the person.
3 **Mobility** Exercise should be kept up until quite late in life. This helps the joints to stay supple so that movement is not cut down. Accidents can be avoided by checking there are no worn stair carpets, loose rugs, or dimly-lit halls.

Mental health

Some people have lively minds at the age of 100. Other people's minds begin to work less well at 60. Just as physical exercise keeps the body healthy, so mental exercise keep the mind active and alert. Taking a university degree or learning about car maintenance or bee-keeping will stimulate the mind.

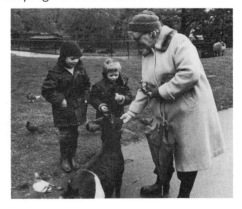

People need to feel loved and useful. This does not stop with old age. Grandparents make good baby-sitters. Small children love to listen to tales of long ago. Some teenagers fear the old. They hide this fear behind cruel jokes. If you are one of these people, remember that the feeling will soon pass. But most young people make excellent companions. They treat elderly people as friends, sharing their troubles and secrets with them.

Finding out:
The work of Age Concern.

Write and ask for details of their work. Do a full project on this.

Questions

1 **The age of retirement is likely to change. Do you think it should be lowered for men, or raised for women? Give reasons for your answer.**
2 **Copy out the figures for where the elderly live.**
3 **Name two normal health problems of growing old and write about two ways in which they can be overcome.**
4 **Have you an elderly person at home? Describe a typical day in their life.**

Handicap and disability

Sometimes, for no reason anyone can understand, a baby is born with a handicap. The baby may be physically disabled – have something wrong with the *body*; or mentally handicapped – have something wrong with the *brain*. In very sad cases, a baby may be born with both physical and mental handicap. This makes life very difficult indeed for the parents.

Attitudes to handicap and disability

People have deep fears about damaged babies. They used to be locked away in institutions so as not to offend our delicate senses. Nowadays, we are less cruel. More and more babies stay at home and in the community. Children are encouraged to attend normal schools, if it is possible. But the words 'cripple' and 'spastic' are still used as insults. Why do you think this is? And what can be done to change people's attitudes?

It is very sad to have a 'less than perfect' baby. The point to understand is that usually nobody is to blame. Not the father, not the mother, not anyone in the family from either side. These things just happen. Parents have to cope with the shock and grief of having a 'less than perfect' baby. The last thing they need is to feel guilty as well.

Mental handicap

This has *nothing* to do with mental illness (p. 60). The two things are quite different. Mental handicap is caused by the brain being physically damaged. This could be at birth, but it can also happen after a road accident (see p. 114). Any really hard blow to the head can damage the brain. When brain cells are destroyed, they cannot mend or heal themselves. The damage is permanent.

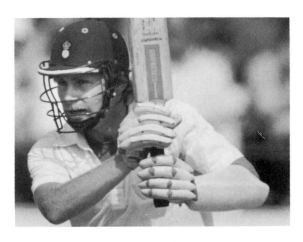

Do you think this player is being over-cautious? Why must you always wear a crash helmet on a motor cycle?

A person who is mentally handicapped is usually very slow at learning. Children can attend special schools where they get the separate attention they need. Some adults can do simple jobs in sheltered workshops – places where they can work at their own speed. Others cannot look after themselves, and have to be cared for in mental homes.

Physical disability

This includes a wide range of things going wrong with the person's *body*. Damaged nerves will stop the muscles working so the person has to use a wheel-chair. Damaged eye-sight, hearing, or speech make learning far more difficult. But this does not mean there is anything wrong with disabled people's minds. They may be very bright indeed. They need to be treated in a cheerful, normal manner, and encouraged to do everything which their disability allows.

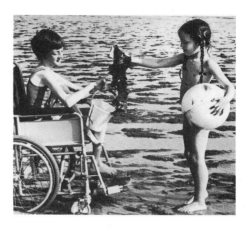

Some ways in which society helps

1. Governments supply financial help. Grants of money include attendance allowance for people who need to be attended (looked after) most of the time; mobility allowance for people who cannot walk but are able to go out; and invalidity pensions for people who cannot work. Large firms are obliged by law to employ a certain number of disabled people.
2. Local councils supply practical help. This includes special housing, special transport, wheelchairs, home nursing, home helps to do the housework, and day centres where disabled people can meet for company.
3. Voluntary organizations give their services free. They rely on donations of money from the public. There are 90,000 registered charities in Britain alone. These include The National Society for Mentally Handicapped Children, The Spastics Society (cerebral palsy), The National Association for Deaf/Blind and Rubella Children, PHAB (The Physically Handicapped and Able-Bodied), and Save the Children.

Can you help?

Community Service Volunteers (CSV) and Task Force are two organizations which need young people to help with community care. Volunteers are expected to work hard, and to learn from the experience. In return, they receive travelling expenses, board and lodging if they move away from home, and – most important – a sense of being wanted and needed, as well as very valuable experience.

Questions

1. **In your own words, explain the difference between physical disability and mental handicap.**
2. **CSV has an Advisory Service which suggests how school and college studies can be linked to helping. At P.E. games for the disabled can be invented. Warning lights for the deaf and bells for the blind can be invented in Science. Can you think of other ways your group could help?**

The caring community

The very young and the very old are dependent upon other people. Babies and small children must be cared for. So must the elderly who become too frail or ill to manage on their own. Other people in the community who need special help are the disabled and handicapped. Some of the services below have already been mentioned in this book.

Home helps are people who come into ordinary homes and do the housework or shopping. Without home helps, many housebound elderly people would have to live in residential homes.

Home nurses work in the community. They visit old or sick people at home to give drugs, change bandages, and do general nursing.

Health visitors are nurses with special training in all family health matters. They give advice on family health problems and how to avoid them.

Chiropodists are trained in foot care. They help old people to stay mobile by treating their foot problems.

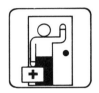

Physiotherapists help disabled people to improve body movement. Their work is very important for young people disabled by road accidents (p. 114).

Occupational therapists show both physically disabled and mentally handicapped people the kinds of occupation (work) best suited to them.

Night attendants watch over very sick or old people during the night.

Ambulance services take people to hospital in emergencies. They also take disabled people to hospital for day treatments.

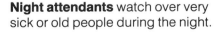

Day centres are for anyone in the community. They particularly cater for old people who meet for company, hot meals, and entertainment.

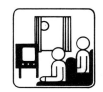

Meals-on-wheels Hot cooked meals are delivered to housebound people in their homes.

Mobile library services lend books to the housebound, and to country people who live too far from their nearest library.

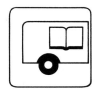

Children's homes look after children who have lost their parents.

Foster homes care for children for a short while only. They give parents a chance to sort out their difficulties before taking their children home.

The NSPCC The National Society for Prevention of Cruelty to Children is concerned with children who are damaged by unhappy parents.

Marriage Guidance Clinics listen to unhappily married people's problems and give advice on how to get over their troubles.

Residential homes These may be specially designed flats or houses for the elderly. They are often run by a warden or a matron.

Geriatric wards are usually in large hospitals. Old people who are very ill receive full nursing care.

Questions

1 **There are far too many community services to be listed here. Think of two which have been left out and write a few lines on each one.**
2 **Write to the local branch of the Red Cross, enclosing a stamped addressed envelope. Do a full project on their work.**
3 **Imagine you have to spend the next three months in bed. Make a list of all the community services you might need.**

A healthy home

Fresh air

In the daylight, plants use up carbon dioxide and give off oxygen. The ultraviolet rays of the sun kill off many germs. Fresh air is good for health as it has more oxygen and less germs in it. Stale air is high in carbon dioxide, moisture, warmth, smoke, or steam. People in stuffy rooms start to feel drowsy. They may yawn, or get a slight headache. They can easily pass on germs.

To **ventilate** a room is to renew or refresh the air. The air in a room needs to be changed frequently, without causing draughts. In hospitals, the air is changed about ten times each hour. Fresh air cuts down the risk of passing on infections. Do you sleep with a window open?

Fresh water

Cold water from the kitchen tap comes straight from the 'mains'. It is fresh and should be used for drinking and cooking food. Water from other taps in the house may have been stored for some time in the tank in the attic. It is more suitable for baths, showers, and so on. From which tap do you fill a glass of water?

Waste water drains into sealed pipes under the ground. Toilets, wash basins, and sinks must be kept thoroughly clean. Remove bits of hair from basins and food scraps from the sink so that the outlet does not get blocked. Check outside drains weekly for rubbish and pour disinfectant down to keep them smelling fresh.

How much water do we use?

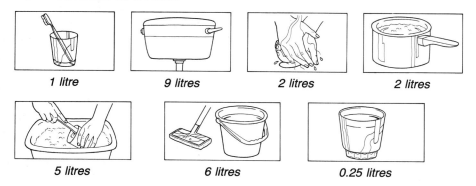

1 litre	9 litres	2 litres	2 litres

5 litres	6 litres	0.25 litres

Lighting

Germs breed best in damp, dark, warm places. Many accidents happen at home because of poor lighting. Dim lights are soothing and give tired eyes a rest. But they should not be used for any kind of close work.

During the day, pull the curtains right back to get as much natural light as possible. In the evenings, artificial light comes from fluorescent tubes or light bulbs. Tubes give a bright sharp light with no shadows – they are useful in kitchens and bathrooms. Dark doorsteps, hallways, and stairs should be kept well lit to avoid accidents. Spotlights are very popular – make sure they shine directly onto your work as this causes the least eye-strain. Students and other people doing close work should rest their eye muscles by staring into the distance every now and then.

Heating

Elderly people and small babies can suffer from **hypothermia** (p. 56). Fires can start in the home if electric flexes are worn, fire-places are left unguarded, or dangerous oil stoves are used. Heating a room without proper ventilation dries the air and makes people cough.

All fires should be checked for safety, and kept well guarded. Dry throats caused by hot rooms can be avoided by putting water containers near sources of heat. The average room temperature for comfort is about 20°C. Elderly people may need extra warmth. Otherwise, the amount of heat in a room is a personal matter. Some people prefer to put on extra woollens and keep the air temperature fairly cool. Air-conditioning, used in hot countries, filters the air and keeps it cool.

The kitchen

This should be well ventilated, well lit, and kept very clean. Food has to be stored, prepared, cooked and the scraps removed in an hygienic way. Work surfaces, sinks, saucepans, cooking utensils, dish cloths, and hands must be thoroughly clean. Food scraps and other waste should be well wrapped and put in a washable bin with a tightly-fitting lid.

Household pests

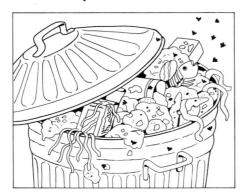

Flies have disgusting habits. They spray food with juice from their mouth parts. When the food is soft, they suck it up and often vomit it back. Germs from their hairy bodies and legs drop onto the food. They live on rotting food near dustbins, or on human and animal waste. They are attracted to it by the smell. Other household pests include cockroaches and silver fish. They can all be killed by using an aerosol spray. Follow the directions on the can. Cover all food first.

Questions

1 **Explain why fresh air is better for health than stale air.**
2 **Why should water from the kitchen tap be used for drinking and cooking?**
3 **Why is it important to have good lighting in the home?**
4 **What should students do to prevent eye-strain?**
5 **Name two important points about heating in the home.**
6 **Explain what might happen if a dustbin does not have a tightly-fitting lid.**

A healthy environment

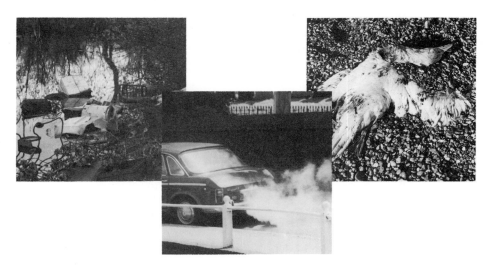

Pollution

Every day, each person produces a great deal of waste. We sweat, we breathe out stale air, we use the toilet – this is personal waste. Household waste includes potato peelings, food wrappings, and dust from the vacuum cleaner. There is also waste from factories, from motor exhausts, from broken-down machines – old cars, old radios, and so on.

To pollute something is to make it dirty and foul. We pollute our environment if we do not get rid of waste safely.

Clean air

City air is polluted by coal and oil being burned in houses and factories, and by exhaust fumes from cars, buses, and aeroplanes. People who live in the country have pink-coloured lungs, but the lungs of town dwellers are often grey with dirt. Air pollution comes next to cigarette smoking as a cause of lung cancer. The lead in petrol can damage a child's brain.

Air pollution is now treated seriously. Strict laws are passed to create 'smokeless zones' in towns. The amount of lead in petrol is to be cut down. More trees, parks, and open spaces help keep the air fresh and clean.

Clean water

Water is polluted if chemical waste from factories and farms is dumped into rivers. Oil spilled from oil-tankers and sewage which is dumped close to the land will pollute the sea. Cholera is a dangerous disease which is carried by water. In very hot countries, all water must be boiled. Cholera can be brought back by infected business travellers or holiday-makers.

Water pumped to the 'mains' in towns is filtered and cleaned. Chlorine is added to it to kill off any germs. Some Water Authorities now add fluoride to the water to prevent tooth decay (p. 40). Strict laws make sure that no untreated waste is dumped in the rivers and seas.

Clean sewage

Sewage is made up of waste from the toilet, bath, wash basin, and kitchen sink. Sewage also comes from factories which may have harmful chemicals in it. All sewage is taken in sealed pipes under the ground to the sewage works. Once the germs are destroyed, the water can than be returned to the rivers. The sludge left over is harmless. It can be used as fertilizer on the land. Most of it is dumped at sea.

Clean housing

Some houses are badly built. They are damp, dark, and difficult to keep clean. Other houses have too many people living in them. Over-crowded and badly-built houses are called slums. Town and country planners are people who decide where new houses, factories, and roads are built. New houses should be convenient to live in – not too far from shops, schools, churches, cinemas, and bus stations. They should also be attractive – with gardens, playgrounds for children, and plenty of grass and trees.

Damp is dangerous in homes as germs feed on the rotting building. This can cause window frames and floors to collapse. Because of the germs, the air in damp houses is not healthy.

Each house must have a damp-proof course (DPC). This is a layer of material which does not allow water to pass through. Cavity walls have a small air space between them. This helps keep out damp, cold air, and noise. It also keeps in warm air – and noise! Noise is now considered a pollutant too. It makes people irritable, and more likely to have accidents. People who live near busy roads or airports need double glazing. This consists of two layers of window glass with an air space between them. It cuts down noise pollution, and keeps in warm air.

Finding out:
More about dry and wet rot.

Write to one of the large manufacturers and ask for leaflets concerning the treatment of dry and wet rot. Do a full project on this.

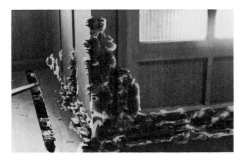

Questions

1 **What is meant by pollution?**
2 **List at least eight kinds of household waste.**
3 **In what ways is air pollution dangerous to health?**
4 **Name two things which are added to town water, and say why.**
5 **Write a short essay on the importance of clean housing.**
6 **Are you a polluter? Do you (a) put bus tickets in the 'used' ticket holder; (b) dump litter in the street rubbish bins; (c) turn the music low late at night; (d) take empty cartons and bottles home after a picnic?**

First aid (1)

Accidents are shocking. They happen so quickly. One minute, everything is normal and the next, someone is badly injured and often in great pain. The suddenness of accidents makes them very frightening. To be of any use, you must try to stay calm. You may be shaking with fright inside, but force yourself to hide it. Remember, panic is catching. The injured person is far more frightened than you.

First aid

The first aider is the person who *first* gives aid. This is usually a close friend or a member of the family. Can you think of the reason why?

All through this book, minor aid for small injuries is included in the relevant section. This section is about very serious injuries which could be a matter of life or death. You may feel a bit squeamish. You may think you couldn't cope. But when someone is terribly injured, you will want to help. You will need to know the right things to do.

First things first

If you are with other people, send someone to call for an ambulance at once. This is very important. If you are not with other people, do not leave the injured person alone. This is equally important. Something much worse could happen to the injured person while you are running for help – which you could have prevented. Stay calm. Think quickly. Start the life-saving checks at once.

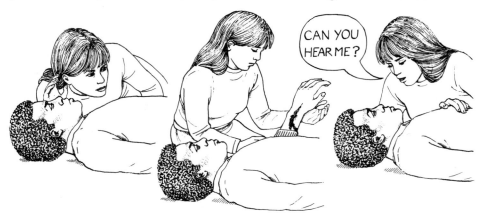

Check for breathing
1   Look to see if the lower chest is moving up and down.
2   Hold the back of your hand close to the mouth and nose to feel for the small draught of air being breathed out.
3   Listen for air being breathed out by putting your ear close to the mouth and nose.
4   Hold a mirror or a piece of cold metal such as a spoon close to the mouth or nose and look to see if breath is steaming it up.
     Do which ever of these things is quickest at the time.

Check for bleeding

This is usually fairly easy. However, the person could be lying on the wound and covering it. It may take a few moments for blood to soak through the clothing before it appears on the ground. Begin the third check at once, remembering to watch out for any blood which appears.

Check the person is conscious

An unconscious person cannot think, speak, or move. He can breathe. Ask questions – 'What is your name? Can you hear me?' Speak quite loudly. A half-conscious person may mumble or make drowsy noises. If he cannot answer in full sentences, he may quickly become unconscious.

The correct order

Breathing? Bleeding? Conscious? This is the correct order in which to do life-saving checks. If breathing stops, brain cells begin to die after four minutes without oxygen. If there is heavy bleeding, the person may very quickly become dangerously ill.

The good first aider remembers to check – Breathing? Bleeding? Conscious? in that order. You also remember to call for an ambulance. All this should not take more than a few moments. Then you set to work.

1 Start the breathing.
2 Stop the bleeding.
3 Make sure the unconscious person does not choke.

Call for an ambulance

Imagine you are the person sent for help. Dial 999. You do not need any money. Emergency services are free. Try not to speak too quickly. Give the address clearly. Add brief directions if it is difficult to find. If you are in a strange place, give the road number or land marks – whatever will be helpful. If you are not near a telephone, stop a passing motorist or knock on the nearest door.

If the person is not too ill and can be moved, it is sometimes quicker to take him straight to a doctor or the hospital. Most people are very helpful, and will immediately offer to drive you both there. 'Call for an ambulance' means take the person to hospital or send for medical help in the quickest way possible.

Finding out:

How quickly you can do the life-saving checks.

Choose a partner and practise in turn. At first, work from the book until you are very quick. Then work from memory. Time yourselves with a stop watch.

Questions

1 **Give your reasons why you think accidents are frightening.**
2 **What are the three life-saving checks? Why are they in this order?**
3 **Write a short account of different ways in which to 'call for an ambulance'.**
4 **Do you think everyone should learn first aid? Give reasons for your answer.**

First aid (2)

Start the breathing

When people faint or collapse, it is not usual for their breathing to stop. Do not rush to give mouth-to-mouth respiration. Always do the checks for breathing first. But accidents such as drowning, suffocation, or drug-overdose (p. 106) can stop breathing. Do not waste time finding out the cause of the accident. Set to work at once. Call for an ambulance.

Check the mouth is empty – not blocked up with seaweed, vomit, or false teeth. Hold the head in both hands and push the jaw upwards and forwards. When the head is in this position, there is no danger of the tongue falling back and blocking the throat. There is a straight clear airway to the lungs. You must learn to do this very quickly. Practise with a friend now.

Mouth-to-mouth respiration

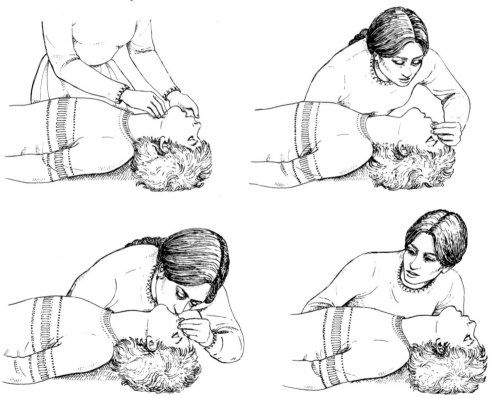

Mouth-to-mouth respiration can *only* be practised on a model. *It is very dangerous to blow air into a person who is breathing normally.*

1 Pinch the nose firmly shut and take a deep breath.
2 Seal your lips over the person's mouth and blow out.
3 Lift your head and watch his chest fall as the air you have blown in comes out.
4 Repeat blowing at your normal rate of breathing, not too fast nor too slow.
5 Go on until help arrives or the person is breathing normally again.

The person may begin to breathe soon after you have started mouth-to-mouth respiration. At first, the breathing may be weak, quick, or gasping. Watch carefully. Be ready to start blowing again if the breathing stops. It may take a few minutes for breathing to settle into a regular, steady pace. Do you remember the breathing rates (p. 34)? Then, very gently, turn the person to the recovery position (p. 170).

Children

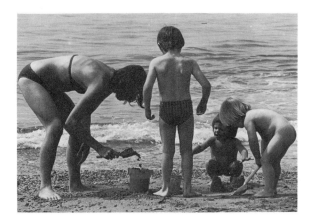

Children have suffocated from putting plastic bags over their heads. As they breathe in, the plastic sticks inside the mouth and nose. It forms an artificial seal and completely blocks off the airway. Toddlers playing in shallow pools fall down and breathe in the water. Babies drown in only a few inches of water if they are left alone in the bath.

1 All plastic bags should be safely disposed of as soon as the goods inside them have been unwrapped.
2 Babies and small children love splashing in water. They should never be left on their own. They must always be carefully watched.

For a baby or very small child, seal your lips right over both the mouth and nose. Remember, you have more air in your lungs than a baby. Blow *gently* and not so *deeply*. It is better to hold the baby in your arms. Keep the head right back with one hand under the jaw.

Questions

1 **Why should you not rush to give mouth-to-mouth respiration if a person collapses? What must you always do first?**
2 **In what way do drug-takers often 'drown'? You may need to turn to page 106 for your answer.**
3 **Name three things you would do to check the airway is clear.**
4 **Copy the diagrams and the instructions for mouth-to-mouth respiration into your book.**
5 **Write about one way in which a small child could stop breathing. What special safety rules would you apply?**
6 **Why should you blow gently and less deeply into a baby's lungs?**

First aid (3)

Stop the bleeding

Blood travels in tubes called arteries and veins. If an artery is cut, the blood spurts high and very fast. If a vein is cut, the blood flows heavily but does not spurt. Heavy bleeding is always serious. It must be stopped at once. The first aid treatment is: *Press down firmly where the blood comes from. Call for an ambulance.*

1 **Raise the bleeding part**
Blood flows more slowly uphill. If an arm or leg is bleeding, raise it quite high. First check that the limb is not lying in an odd position. This could mean a bone is broken and then the limb must not be moved. Having raised the bleeding part, rest it comfortably on a stool, a garden wall, or on top of your folded coat.

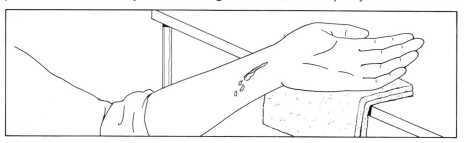

2 **Press down firmly on the pad**
Make a pad from anything – a scarf, tie, or handkerchief. Put the pad on top of the wound and press down firmly. Do not be afraid of hurting the person. Do not worry about germs or dirt. Keep pressing down for at least ten minutes. You must stop the bleeding. Keep the pad absolutely still.

3 **Press the edges of the wound together**
Some cuts are long and wide. The edges will have to be stitched together in hospital. With the fingers of both hands, press the skin forward so that the edges come together. Keep pressing down firmly.

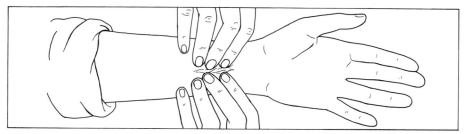

4 **Tie a bandage over the pad**
While you wait for the bleeding to stop, keep chatting calmly to the injured person. This is a great comfort. At the same time, keep a look-out for someone to call for an ambulance. If you have shoe-laces or a belt, use this as a bandage to tie around the pad. Try not to make jolting movements. Do not lift up the pad to see if bleeding has stopped. Either of these can start the bleeding again. If blood does come through the pad, put another one on top and press down firmly for another ten minutes.

Very important points

1 If there is something sticking out of the wound, such as a piece of glass, leave it there. *You must not try to pull it out.* You will cause far more bleeding and perhaps a far more serious injury.
2 Press down on *either side* of the wound to help stop the bleeding.
3 *Nothing by mouth.* Never give a person who is bleeding heavily anything to eat or drink. When they get to hospital, they may need an anaesthetic (a drug to make them unconscious). If there is food or water in the stomach, the person may vomit and choke during the operation.

Bleeding from the ear or nose after a blow on the head

Any hard blow on the head can damage the brain. This is very serious as it could lead to mental handicap (p. 156). The person may be briefly **concussed** (knocked out) and come round in a short while. Do *not* try to stop any bleeding from the nose or ear. Call an ambulance immediately. Turn the person to the **recovery position** (see p. 170).

Treatment for a simple nose bleed

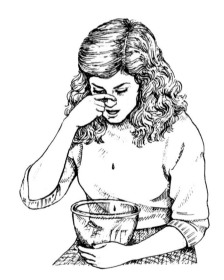

1 Sit on a chair near the sink, or with a bowl in your lap.
2 Put your head forward and down to stop blood trickling back to the throat.
3 Pinch the nose firmly about a third of the way down for ten minutes.
4 Movement will stop the blood clotting. Don't talk. Swallow gently. Breathe through the mouth.
5 Sit quietly for a while afterwards and do not blow your nose.

Finding out:
Your first-aid skills on this unit.

Working in twos, practise how to stop bleeding.

Questions

1 **Copy out the first-aid treatment for heavy bleeding.**
2 **How could you tell if bleeding was from an artery or a vein?**
3 **Explain why the bleeding part should be raised if possible.**
4 **Turn to page 38 and re-read how blood clots. Why should you not make any jolting movements when bandaging the wound?**
5 **What would you do if there was a pair of scissors sticking out of the wound?**
6 **A person who is bleeding heavily begs you for a drink of water. Explain, very clearly, why you would refuse to give it.**

First aid (4)

Unconscious?

The first aider's work is to make sure the unconscious person is breathing. Then you must make sure they *go on* breathing. Loosen any tight clothing at the neck and waist. If they are lying on their back, the tongue can fall down the throat and cut off breathing. If they are sick, the vomit can slide down into the lungs and choke them. Turn the person to the recovery position to stop these things happening. Call for an ambulance.

The recovery position

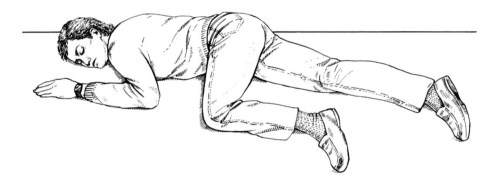

It may seem difficult to turn a heavy person over. It is not. Kneel down at their right side. Tuck one hand under their left knee. Grasp their left shoulder with your other hand. Then, using the person's own weight, you can roll them over towards you. Turn their head sideways and slightly upwards. Move one arm up and out so that the body weight is comfortable. Tuck a smooth cloth under the head. Cover the person with a blanket.

    The recovery position is the safest way to place anyone who is seriously injured. However, if there are signs of broken bones (p. 28) the person must *not* be moved. Make sure the breathing passage is clear by tilting the head right back, and holding it there. Never give anything to drink, even to a half-conscious person. If the throat muscles are not working properly, there can be no swallowing. The water will almost certainly go down into the lungs and cause drowning (p. 34).

Shock

To most people, shock means being badly shaken-up after an accident. But to doctors, nurses, and first aiders, shock means something far more serious. Shock means a *dangerous state* in which the whole body is *very ill*. This can happen after heavy bleeding. The person collapses and must be given new blood, urgently.

Signs of shock

The person's colour changes. Brown or black people go a dark blue-grey. White or yellow people go a dirty pale grey. The skin is cold, clammy, and damp with chilly sweat. Breathing is weak or gasping. The pulse is weak and faster than normal.

The person's behaviour changes too, becoming restless or confused. People in shock may not know where they are, or what has happened. They may insist they are quite well. They may try to get up. *They must not do this. A person in shock must lie down.*

To prevent shock

1 Stop any heavy bleeding.
2 Lie the person down, with the head low and the feet raised. This helps the blood flow back to the brain.
3 Turn the person's head to the side so that there is no risk of choking if they become unconscious. Be very gentle in your movements.
4 Keep the person warm, but not hot. Cover with one blanket; two if it is a cold day. Never use hot-water bottles. They can increase shock.
5 Comfort the person and soothe away fears. This is a very important part of the first aider's work, *especially for shock*. A sudden collapse is always frightening. When a person is restless, anxious, and upset, *shock gets worse*. Begin to talk to the person as soon as you start helping. (It's not *what* you say that matters as much as the *way* you say it. Sound calm and confident: The ambulance is on its way . . . You'll see the children are picked up from school . . . There's nothing to worry about . . . You won't leave the person . . . , and so on.) Always remember a shocked person may be in great pain. Be as gentle, careful, and comforting as you possibly can.

Finding out:
Your first-aid skills on this unit.

Working in twos, practise turning someone to the recovery position. Move your partner slowly and gently. Then practise the five steps in treatment for shock.

Questions

1 **What is always the danger when a person becomes unconscious?**
2 **Explain clearly why the recovery position is the safest for an injured person.**
3 **What is the one type of injury when you would *not* use the recovery position?**
4 **Explain what is meant by 'shock',**
5 **Describe the symptoms of shock.**
6 **Write a brief essay, discussing the best ways to prevent shock.**

First aid (5)

How to treat burns

Burned skin stays burning for a short while after you have hurt it. This is rather like a boiled egg which goes on cooking when it is first taken out of water. The first aider's job is to stop skin getting more damaged. Do this by putting the burned part into cold water immediately. The first aid treatment is: *cold water on the burn for ten minutes, urgently.*

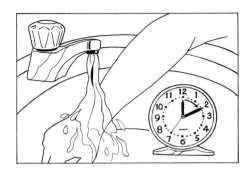

Stopping the pain

Cold water on burned skin also stops the pain. But the burned part must be covered in cold water for the full ten minutes. Think how long it takes to cool a hard-boiled egg! Always time the cooling process. Gently pat the burned part dry. Cover with a clean dry dressing to stop germs getting in. Never put creams, lotions, or ointments on a burn.

For large burns

Imagine little Susan comes running into the room. Her skirt is on fire. What should you do? Pick up the nearest large cloth – rug, blanket, or coat. Wrap it tightly around her so that no air can get in. Fire cannot burn without the oxygen which is in air. As soon as you cut off the air, the fire stops.

1   Call for an ambulance immediately.
2   Carry Susan to the bathroom and put her gently into the bath.
3   Half fill the bath with cool, not cold, water. Putting a badly-burned person into cold water causes shock, which is very dangerous.
4   Make sure the whole of the burned side is covered with water.
5   Support Susan's head. If she became unconscious, she might slide down and drown.
6   Stay with Susan till help arrives. If she is fully conscious, give her small repeated sips of water. This is important as body fluids escape from burned broken skin. They must be replaced.

All people suffering from large burns must be taken to hospital as soon as possible. The only time the first aider gives water is for burns, and for outdoors cold exposure.

Heat stroke

Heat stroke happens in very hot countries, especially when the air is humid (full of water). The person cannot lose body heat by sweating. They are over-heated by the sun or hot air around them. They have a very high temperature; their skin is burning hot, red, and dry. Their mind may be confused. They may have a splitting headache and they can quickly become unconscious.

1 Call an ambulance immediately.
2 Help the person into the shade and start to cool them down.
3 If possible, lower them gently into a bath of cool, not cold, water.
4 If not, remove their clothes and sponge them with plenty of tepid water.
5 Stay with them till help arrives. Keep on cooling them down, slowly.

Outdoors cold exposure

For frost bite: Never rub the 'bitten' frozen part. This breaks open the blood tubes under the skin and makes the damage much worse. The frozen part must be warmed, slowly.
For very cold water: If you fall in, stay still and call for help. Do not try to swim in icy water or you will lose what is left of your body heat. Remember, it is as important to wear really warm clothes in a boat as it is to wear a life-jacket.

The first aid treatment for outdoors exposure is:

1 Get the person to safety and hospital as quickly as possible.
2 A strong healthy young person can be put in a bath of really warm water.
3 A very ill, weak person must be warmed slowly.
4 Hot drinks can be given for all cold chilling *if the person is fully conscious. Nothing by mouth* otherwise.

The first-aid box

The first-aid box must have a child-proof lock, or be kept in a locked cupboard. It is useful for minor injuries which can be treated at home.

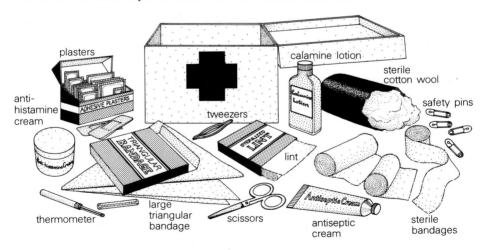

Questions

1 **What is the first-aid treatment for burns?**
2 **What two things does this treatment do?**
3 **Why should water be given to a person with burns?**
4 **Explain what is meant by heat stroke.**
5 **What should you do if you fall into really icy water, and why?**
6 **Copy out the contents of the first-aid box into your book.**

Further work on Chapter 5

1 Visit an antenatal clinic and make notes on what you observe.

2 Write a short essay about Down's Syndrome.

3 What is meant by 'amniocentesis'? Write a short account of what might happen if the foetus is found to be handicapped.

4 Unhappy couples may have a baby to help patch up their marriage. Do you think this might be helpful, or not? Give reasons for your answer.

5 Write to your local branch of the National Society for the Prevention of Cruelty to Children – the NSPCC. Do a full project on their work.

6 Explain why couples should not be upset if they do not conceive immediately after they stop using family planning.

7 Write a full account of the things which can harm an unborn baby. Then explain why a planned baby is less likely to undergo these risks.

8 From the text, copy out the list of checks which happen to a mother at the antenatal clinic.

9 From the text on page 150, copy out the averages for (a) new-born babies and (b) toddlers.

10 Find out about the work of welfare officers. Do a project on the ways in which they help children.

11 What clues will a doctor be looking for when taking note of a person's general appearance at a complete health check-up?

12 If possible, visit a mobile health unit. Write to your local health education office for details of when this can be arranged.

13 There is a general idea that families nowadays do not care for their elderly. Write a short account of why this is not so.

14 Make arrangements to visit a local Residential Home for the Elderly. Study the various ways in which the staff help elderly people to keep active and alert. Why do you think this is important?

15 Write an account of attitudes towards handicap and disability.

16 If possible, arrange to visit your local branch of PHAB or any organization which helps the disabled. Do a project on their work. Perhaps you might be interested in offering your help?

17 Young people suffer brain damage and become mentally handicapped from accidents on the road (p. 114). In what ways do the laws concerning seat belts and crash helmets attempt to protect them?

18 If possible, arrange for a fully-trained first aider to give a demonstration of mouth-to-mouth respiration to your group. A staff member from St John's Ambulance or the Red Cross may be able to help.

19 Do a full project on first aid. Contact your local branch of St John's Ambulance and ask for information and help.

Index